Outcome Measures in Home Care

Volume I
Research

Lynn T. Rinke, MS, RN, Editor

Director
Division of Accreditation for Home Care
and Community Health
National League for Nursing

Pub. No. 21-2194

National League for Nursing • New York

ISBN 0-88737-378-X

Manufactured in the United States of America.

CONTENTS

PART 3: THE RECORD AS A DATA SOURCE

PART 4: COMMUNITY-BASED DEMONSTRATIONS

PART 5: INSTRUMENT DEVELOPMENT

PREFACE

Home Care Outcomes: Focus on Research

The 1980s have been a period of great change and tumult in the health care delivery system in the United States. As nursing confronts all at once a health care crisis precipitated by the introduction of the Medicare prospective payment system for hospital care, the realization that public health measures and life-style changes are the major variables to improving health status, and an aging population with chronic health problems, we are acknowledging the failure of the bio-medical, institutionally based health care delivery paradigm. The current and future variations on the perennial problems of the cost of, quality of, and access to health care cannot be met with the old medical model. A community-based nursing paradigm offers great potential for efficacious solutions to both old and new problems in health care delivery.

This anthology marks the introduction of a new series of publications from the National League for Nursing. The series will focus on issues germane to the delivery of community-based care services. Since nursing care is, and has been for a century, the cornerstone of in-home health care, the profession needs to assume leadership in ushering in the new paradigm for health care delivery in this country. This anthology aims to promote nursing leadership in home care research by providing a single reference to the classic and current literature addressing outcomes in home care.

The second publication in this series will address initiatives from the service sector in defining and measuring home care outcomes that have been carried out by nurses in a variety of public, private, and voluntary home care agencies. The third volume will be a monograph, a meta-analysis of the work published in the first two books, with a focus on the public policy interests in home care outcomes.

RESEARCHING HOME CARE OUTCOMES

Health status outcomes are finally receiving sincere attention in the professional health care community, although Avedis Donabedian, the author of the first chapter in this volume, introduced the concept more than 20 years ago. And although professional home care is almost a century old practice in this country, it is only recently that we have started to give serious attention to the health outcomes realized by such services.

The pieces reprinted in this anthology represent a broad variety of literature relevant to the issues in researching home care outcomes. The seemingly disparate perspectives represented in this collection reflect the current chaos in the field as practitioners and researchers attempt to grapple with the issues of defining and measuring the outcomes of home health care.

Part 1 commences with a general introduction by Donabedian, addressing "Some Basic Issues in Evaluating the Quality of Health Care." Although an entire anthology of Donabedian's works on this issues could be amassed, this particular piece not only describes the major tenets of his classic work but also represents his ideas as directed to the nursing community. The next two pieces by Hegyvary and Haussmann and by Horn and Swain summarize the seminal nursing research on outcome measures. Although neither paper addresses home care, any discussion of nursing research and health outcomes would be incomplete without acknowledging the contributions of these investigators. Furthermore, these research reports might serve as useful foundations, by extension, for developing outcome research in home care. The final piece in this section, by Januska, Engle, and Wood, is the only previously unpublished manuscript in the anthology. We have printed "Status of Quality Assurance in Public Health Nursing" as presented at the 1976 Annual Meeting of the American Public Health Association as a service to the profession; often referenced, this piece is a classic on the state of the art of quality assurance for community-based nursing services through the mid-1970s.

Part 2 includes two pieces addressing maternal-child health home care services. As a nurse researcher, Barkauskas pioneered efforts to document health outcomes related to public health nurse visits. Brooten and her colleagues, medical researchers, document positive outcomes for services similar to those described by Barkauskas but targeted to a specific high-risk population.

The two papers in Part 3 reflect a major methodological challenge in documenting outcomes—using patient care records as a primary data source. Day's report reflects the issues identified by Koerner's examination of the validity of the documentation of community health nurses.

Part 4 consists of a single article, the introduction to a meta-analysis of 13 federally funded community care demonstration projects. It is offered as a summary of the 13 demonstration projects, and also addresses various structural, process, and outcome measures significant to community-based care initiatives.

Part 5 deals with the development of tools for measuring the health outcomes of home care. Choi, Josten, and Christensen's work on the Family Coping Index is unique in addressing the family as the unit of care. Padilla and Grant use a measure of quality of life—a nonmedical variable—as an outcome measure for cancer nursing. The final selection by Lalonde represents a portion of a current work-in-progress to develop reliable and valid outcome measures for home care. This piece also includes a section on reliability and validity that will provide the reader with a useful review of concepts for evaluating the outcomes presented throughout this book.

We anticipate that this anthology will contribute significantly to the current discussion on home care outcomes. We hope it will stimulate timely nursing research on the effectiveness of health care in the community—a virtually autonomous nursing practice domain.

—Lynn T. Rinke, MS, RN

Part 1

REFLECTIONS

Some Basic Issues in Evaluating the Quality of Health Care

Avedis Donabedian

Quality care has been a central objective of the nursing profession, and the means to assure it a constant preoccupation. A renewal of research in nursing care reveals some most imaginative approaches to evaluating quality, notably an early emphasis on patient progress and an insistence that the social, psychological, and ethical dimensions of care are central to the notion of quality. Even though I shall speak of "medical" care, and draw my examples largely from the literature of medicine, the issues that I shall raise cut across the boundaries of professional parochialism to include us all.

THE DEFINITION OF QUALITY

A small number of basic issues lie close to the heart of assessment. The first issue has to do with defining the concept of quality so that we can have a common framework for discourse and investigation. To help us arrive at this happy state, I have constructed a cubical structure which is shown in Figure 1.

On one side of this cube, we recognize that there are many aspects to the concept of "health." In this instance, we have distinguished three: physical-physiological function, psychological function, and social function. There is nothing sacred or fixed about this simple-minded classification. You might, quite properly, use a different one. What is important is to recognize that the manner in which we conceive of health and of our responsibility for it, makes a fundamental difference to the concept of quality and, as a result, to the methods that we use to assess and assure the quality of care.

Another side of the diagram shows levels of aggregation of the subjects of care. Here, we make an important distinction between a "patient," who has already gained access to some care, and a "person," who may or may not have done so. Under each of these primary categories there is a further distinction between the individual and the aggregate of individuals.

FIGURE 1
Level and Scope of Concern as Factors in the Definition of Quality

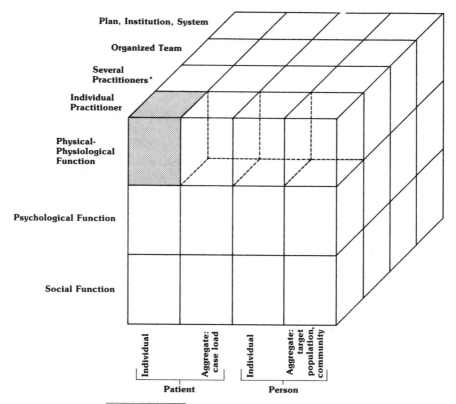

* Of the same profession or of different professions

The third side of our cubical figure shows levels of aggregation and organization of the providers of care. The initial level of concern is with the care provided by an individual practitioner without reference to who else may be involved in the care of any particular subject, whether it be an individual or aggregate. From here one moves on to include the contributions of more than one practitioner, in the same or different professions, who may be providing care concurrently, as individuals, or jointly, as a team. At even higher levels of aggregation we are concerned with the performance of institutions or programs, and of the health care system as a whole.

Let us now examine some of the implications of this formulation.

So far, studies of the quality of care have focused on the clinical management of the individual patient by the individual practitioner; and the main object of concern, more so in medicine than in nursing, has been on physical and physiological function. We have already suggested that the definition of health can be enlarged to include other aspects of an individual's performance. But such an extension cannot occur simply because the researcher or administrator wills it. It can be legitimate only to the extent that there is a social consensus that the scope of professional competence and responsibility embraces these areas of function. A corollary is that such extensions cannot be made unilaterally by health professionals, since they impinge on what consumers expect, want, or are willing to accept. But professionals must bear the burden of leadership in such matters.

From the primordial cell in our framework, shown by the shaded area in Figure 1, we can move outward to include more and more of our cubical structure. As we do so, new considerations enter the picture, which modify our notions of quality and render its assessment increasingly difficult. When more than one practitioner are involved in the provision of care, we are confronted with the problem of assessing the separate and joint contributions of each. As care becomes more highly organized, attributes such as "continuity," "coordination," and, even, "teamhood" become important constituents of the concept of quality. But these attributes are difficult to define and even more difficult to measure, so that their contribution to quality has remained largely untested. There is little doubt, however, that these and other properties of the system that provides health care can influence the achievement of health care objectives and, for that reason, have a legitimate place in the definition of quality when such systems are the objects of assessment.

The concept of quality is also altered by the level of aggregation of the subjects of care. The major attribute that emerges when we move from "patient" to "person" is that of access. The major issue that surfaces when we compare care for the individual to care for the collectivity is that of resource allocation. Access and resource allocation are, themselves, interrelated, since they both have to do with who gets care, of what kind, and how much. These questions are, in turn, related to a number of deeper policy issues, including equity and the cost-effect relationships in allocative efficiency.

When the care of each individual patient is considered, it is generally assumed that resources are virtually limitless, and that all that is likely to be beneficial will be done. But, in real life, resources are limited, so that more care for the few is often at the expense of some care for many. That this is true for target populations is generally recognized. But we should also remember that each practitioner is constantly called upon to partition among those who depend upon him or her for care, that most precious of all resources, the practitioner's own time and attention. Thus, it is reasonable to argue that not only the program as a whole, but also each practitioner should be judged not only by the care given each patient, but also by the manner in which a total population or a case load is managed.

We see, through these few examples, that the concept of quality changes in context as we move from one domain to another within the frame of reference of which our cubical figure is a crude representation. To some extent, this need not give us concern, since what happens is an extension and enrichment of the concept of quality, as it acquires additional envelopes of meaning. But that is only part of what takes place. There is also the potential for conflict among the competing objectives that are introduced. Chief among these is the conflict between the practitioner's responsibility to the individual as compared to the responsibility to an aggregate. This problem has always been with us, but as care has become organized and its financing collectivized, the problem has become more difficult to ignore. Increasingly, the practitioner has been placed in the difficult position of being required to pursue the private interests of each patient with due regard to the interests of all patients. The standard of behavior that reconciles the two interests is not as clear as that which assumes exclusive commitment to each patient.

Whether a case with syphilis is to be reported or not, whether it is justifiable to engage in activities the chief purpose of which is learning or teaching, whether it is proper to curtail care to the individual in order to enhance access to greater numbers, whether it is justifiable to increase costs to the individual in order to reduce them for the financing program: all these are examples of the conflict between the responsibility of the practitioner to the patient as an individual and to society as a collectivity.

Thus, as we move from our concern with the evaluation of the technical management of health states at the individual level to the social management of these states at the collective level, we are in danger of losing our initial innocence. Until then, we had thought that quality could be built up, from low levels to high, by increments, each of which contributed positively to the total. Now, we are no longer certain: and it looks as if in order to provide better care for all we may have to provide less good care to some. The concept of quality, no longer benignly seductive, looks us sternly in the face and offers a moral dilemma.

THE OBJECT OF EVALUATION

Having established a frame of reference, which I hope you will find useful, we are ready to move on to the second basic issue before us: that of the proper object of evaluation.

In her seminal paper on "Approaches to the Quality of Hospital Care," the late Mindel Sheps concluded that

> the main techniques used in appraisals of hospital quality can be divided into:
>
> • The examination of prerequisites or desiderata for adequate care.
>
> • Indexes of elements of performance.
>
> • Indexes of the effects of care.
>
> • Qualitative clinical evaluations. [1]

As I pondered this classification, it seemed to me that the last and second of these categories were similar, and that if they were combined a simple classification would emerge; namely: "structure," "process," and "outcome." [2]

This simple trichotomy has proven useful to many, so that the words "structure," "process," and "outcome" have become part of the everyday language of our field. More importantly, this formulation has prompted attempts at modification and extension, the most important of which, to my knowledge, is that of De Geyndt, who has distinguished five "approaches" to assessing the quality of care: "content," "process," "structure," "outcome," and "impact." [3]

The academician can have a field day comparing the two classifications and teasing out the logical relationships between the two. But it seems to me that the two classifications are fully congruent, and that the differences in detail, important though these are, have arisen from a shift in position within the frame of reference which we took some pains to construct at the very outset. As one moves from concern with the care provided by one practitioner to that provided by aggregates or organized groupings of practitioners, the process of care appears to become readily differentiated into two components, one of which is what De Geyndt refers to as "content." The other component, which could be called "configuration," but which De Geyndt names "process," includes properties such as continuity, coordination, sequencing, and even that yet undefined attribute or set of attributes that we have referred to as "teamhood." Similarly, as one moves from concern for individual patients to concern for a population, the logical category of "outcome" might bifurcate into "end results," which describe states of individuals, and "impacts," which describe states of populations taken in the whole. These relationships are schematically represented in Figure 2.

My purpose in reviewing these developments has not been to reassure ourselves that "structure-process-outcome" endures, and all's well with the world. On the contrary, I believe that the apparent usefulness and the seductive simplicity of this formulation can readily lead to its abuse, so that it becomes an obstacle rather than a help. This happens, for example, where there is insistence on assigning primacy to one of the elements over another. This has generally taken the form of a contest for preeminence between process and outcome; one or the other is held to be supreme. In fact, the question which of the triad is primary and which subsidiary arises from the context (or frame of reference) for evaluation, rather than from the elements themselves.

In the particular context of evaluating the performance of practitioners in caring for individual patients, I have felt it more reasonable (I could have said, "more relevant to the object of analysis") to give primacy to the process of care, and to consider structural attributes and outcomes as indirect measures, or evidence, of the quality of the process, on the assumption that certain attributes of structure are conducive to certain levels of performance and these, in turn, are conducive to the achievement of certain states of the patient. In another context, outcome might be the primary object of analysis, and process or structure "proxy measures" of outcome. Few, if any, have championed the primacy of structure in evaluations of the quality of medical care, but I can imagine situations in which the evaluation of structure might well be the primary focus of interest, and that process and outcome might serve as proxy measures of structure.

Besides the observation that each of structure, process, or outcome can serve as the primary focus of inquiry, depending on the context, one observes that aspects of structure, process, and outcome often flow into each other in a linear

FIGURE 2
Classifications of Approaches to Assessing the Quality of Health Care as Proposed by Donabedian and by De Geyndt

Classification by Donabedian	Synthesis of the Two Classifications	Classification by De Geyndt
STRUCTURE	Structure	STRUCTURE
PROCESS	Content	CONTENT
	Configuration	PROCESS
OUTCOME	End Result	OUTCOME
	Impact	IMPACT

Sources: A. Donabedian, "Evaluating the Quality of Medical Care," *Milbank Memorial Fund Quarterly,* 44 (July 1966), Part 2, 166–206; and Willy De Geyndt, "Five Approaches to Assessing the Quality of Care," *Hospital Administration,* 15 (Winter 1970), 21–42.

or branched chain of ends and means.[4] Hence, we hear of intervening categories such as "procedural end points,"[5] "proximate outcomes," "intermediate outcomes," and "remote" or "ultimate outcomes." Again, what segment of the chain is examined, and which are the means and which the ends, depends on the context. This formulation and the presence of intervening processes and states offer the happy prospect of reconciliation among what seem to be opposing positions; so much so that I am tempted to propose that very often we are concerned not with the evaluation of "process" or of "outcome" but with something in between, which we might, rather tongue-in-cheek, designate as either "procome" or "outcess."[6]

Moving from theory to practice, I am convinced that we do not, at present, know enough to base any program of quality assessment and assurance exclusively on any one of structure, process, or outcome. We need to use all three simultaneously. Furthermore, we need to design our system to give information about the relationships among the three, so that we can begin to understand what aspects of structure help the attainment of desired attributes of process and the extent to which these latter contribute to desired outcomes. A thorough grasp of these three relationships is the only valid basis for corrective or preventive action to safeguard quality.

THE EVALUATION OF OUTCOME

The evaluation of outcome is particularly attractive because it satisfies the eminently reasonable argument that all the health care in the world is for naught unless it makes some impact on health. Moreover, most people agree on what are desired health outcomes, so that the criteria enjoy a great deal of face validity. Finally, health outcomes have an integrative property that seems to solve many of the problems of quality assessment. At the level of the individual patient, outcomes represent the result of the efforts of all those who have been involved in the patient's care. At the population level, health outcomes represent the operation of the health services system as a whole, including the effects of access, resource allocation, external benefits, and the conformity of professional performance to professional norms. Thus, we seem to have summarized in one measure all that we need to know.

Alas, as we shall see, the use of outcomes in quality assessment also suffers from serious handicaps, some of which are not easily remedied. At the very outset, the agreement on what are desired outcomes begins to crumble when the concept of health is enlarged to include psychological and social health. For example, it is not at all clear that contentment and conformity are, in all instances, preferable to tension or rebellion. Nor is it universally accepted that some life, no matter how impoverished, is preferable to no life at all. Agreement on such fundamental social values becomes a prerequisite to the use of outcomes for assessment at certain levels of analysis.

Even when there is less ambiguity concerning the desirability of the end state itself, it is necessary to establish that it is achievable by good health care in any given situation. A corollary is that the outcome in question is relevant to the goals of the health professionals as defined by themselves, by the health care system of which they are a part, or by society at large.

Additional difficulties arise from the fact that outcomes are time-dependent in two ways. First, the consequences of care may take some time to become apparent, which makes such outcomes unsuitable for assessment in the short run. A second, more fundamental, feature is that outcomes have a time dimension incorporated into them. Certain modifications in health status are temporary, whereas others are of long duration. It is necessary to include these differences in any accounting of the consequences of care.[7] The system of accounting must also be one that permits us to measure in equivalent terms mortality as well as varying kinds and severities of morbidity and dysfunction. The impact of mortality is generally measured as the period elapsed between the time of death and either the time of expected death, or some arbitrary age which limits the human life span. The specification and measurement of states of dysfunction is more difficult; and most difficult has been the problem of weighting the states of dysfunction, so that a single measure of health status can be constructed.[8]

The ultimate measure of the success or failure of the health care system may well be the survival table, but not in years alone. It is necessary to obtain some measure of the quality of life during the increment of years that is conferred by the ministrations of the health professions. But, a consideration of what makes life worthwhile raises the most fundamental issues of the human personality and of the place of the individual in society. When we assess the failure or success of the patient-practitioner transaction, we must recognize that each person decides what in life is worthwhile, and at what point mere survival has ceased to be meaningful. At the collective level, it should be possible to embody in a measure of survival the general values to which society subscribes. At this level, what determines the quality of care is necessarily dependent on what constitutes the quality of life.

Assuming that the problems of measuring outcomes have been solved, a final obstacle remains, which is assigning the place and degree of responsibility for the outcomes observed. This is the problem of attribution. It arises partly from the multiplicity of factors that can influence health and partly from imperfections in our knowledge of the precise relationship between each factor and health. Among the factors that influence the outcomes of care are many over which the health care system has either no jurisdiction or no influence. It follows that the operation of such factors must be neutralized through rigorous research design. Thus, the identification and equalization of risk factors is a necessary precondition to the assessment of outcomes. The difficulties of attribution can also be reduced by the choice of a battery of proximate outcomes that are reasonably specific for each of the conditions for which care is being provided. A dual benefit would be the result: a system of management by objectives that would also lend itself to concurrent monitoring and retrospective review. Seeing the magnitude of the advantage that would ensue, it is surprising that this approach to the control and assessment of care has not received a higher place on the research agenda.

THE EVALUATION OF PROCESS

The evaluation of process is, in some ways, a counterpart to the assessment of outcome. Here we have the advantage of immediate or early feedback; but the major disadvantage is that the validity of the criteria and standards is much more subject to serious question. The unconfirmed, or imperfectly substantiated, validity of process criteria corresponds, in a way, to the attribution problem in the assessment of outcomes, for it questions whether any given components of clinical management have contributed to desired or undesired states of health. There are two kinds of validity, however, and only the first has to do with the relationship between elements of process and attributes of outcome. Questions concerning it arise because of imperfections in the health sciences. If this is true of the management of physical and physiological health, it is even more so in the realm of psychological and social health, where our science is relatively rudimentary and largely untested.

The first kind of validity, that concerning the causal relationships between process and outcome, is conceptually separable from another, which deals with the norms and conventions of professional behavior. Here, we do not ask whether our science is any good, but whether available knowledge has been properly applied in the management of the dysfunction states for which the practitioner has a legitimate responsibility. This involves (1) the proper specification of the health situation, which is called "diagnosis"; (2) the decision to intervene or not; (3) the choice of the objectives of intervention; (4) the choice of the modalities, methods, and techniques that are meant to achieve these objectives; and (5) the properly skillful execution of these techniques. Under this formulation, the quality of care is redefined, simply, as normative behavior. But since the emergence of norms is often dependent on the prior validation of the contribution of process to outcome, and where norms are not clearly established, the judgment concerning quality must remain correspondingly uncertain.

If quality can be redefined as normative behavior, the study of the derivation, structure, prevalence, and penetrance of norms must be an important part of the research in quality assessment. A recent study by Hare and Barnoon illustrates both the problems and potentials of such research.[9] The investigators selected six diagnostic categories that were considered important in the practice of internists. A comprehensive set of "criteria" was constructed which listed all the procedures that might be carried out in the management of each condition. Samples of internists in different parts of the United States were then asked to indicate how important each of these items was in the management of each condition. This enabled the investigators to rank the items by importance. Subsequently, records kept by each physician were examined in order to determine how frequently each of the items in the lists of criteria were performed in actual practice. As a result it was possible to rank the items by frequency of performance. A comparison of the two rankings, one by perceived importance and one by frequency of performance, among internists in different areas of the United States showed that physicians agreed on what they thought was important and were also similar in the way they practiced. This is good news to those who would see quality as normative behavior. Unfortunately, the investigators also found that there was no correlation between the ranking by importance and that by frequency.

It is easy to find fault with the methods and rationale of this study. In particular, one might question whether perceived importance and practiced frequency are congruent concepts. It would also be facile to conclude, assuming the findings are accepted as reasonably valid, that physicians do not practice what they know to be good, and that, therefore, the quality of care is bad. An alternative explanation is that, in actual practice, physicians must respond to a clinical situation of such detailed specificity that it is very imperfectly represented by a broad diagnostic category, even when reasonably large numbers of cases are reviewed. Moreover, actual practice represents an adaptation to a multiplicity of partially conflicting goals at least some of which are socially legitimate. If so, it would mean that the listings of all the things that it is good to do in the management of specified conditions represent the dictates of science essentially unmodified by considerations of relative priorities, of patient acceptability, of resource allocation, and of benefits relative to costs. In contrast, the practice of "good" physicians in "favorable" settings would represent a more socially relevant standard of care. Having arrived at this hypothesis, it would be tragically dangerous to stop, and to use it as a justification for accepting prevalent practice as the standard of care. This is emphatically not the intent. On the contrary, the intent is to stimulate conceptual development and empirical research to determine what styles and strategies of care are optimal in terms of multiple objectives at the individual and collective levels. But, before we pursue this subject further, it would be useful to consider in more detail some alternative approaches to the assessment of process.

In a paper that describes the pioneering studies of the quality of medical care in the Health Insurance Plan of Greater New York, Henry Makover[10] quotes an editorial from the *Lancet,* as follows:

> The other day an experienced physician was asked what criteria he would apply in judging the efficiency of a hospital; what relative importance

he would attach to the qualifications of the staff, the ratio of beds to nurses, the adequacy of special departments, the catering, the facilities for reablement, and the various other items on which inspecting authorities commonly make notes. He replied, "I should not inquire into any of these things. I should simply go into the wards, select six patients, and find out precisely what had been done for them, and the care that they had received, since the day of their admission." This wise answer has implications beyond even the hospital services, for it embodies the truth that any kind of machinery, however ingenious, is but a means to an end.[11]

In this same tradition was the subsequent work under the leadership of Mildred Morehead, except that almost exclusive reliance had to be placed on the hospital record, with all its recognized limitations as a source of information.[12] This deficiency, which could be rectified only in part by interviewing the attending physicians, was counterbalanced, however, by what I believe was the fundamental soundness of the basic idea: that the judgment of quality (in this context) must depend on a total assessment of the total care of a patient who presents as a problem for diagnosis and management; and that the assessment must reflect the best judgment of a mature and skilled physician charged with reviewing each case. Unfortunately, in hands less skillful than Morehead's, the reliability of such judgments was found to be so low that the entire procedure has fallen into disrepute.

THE CRITERIA APPROACH

The alternative method that has been proposed originated in the pioneering work of Paul Lembcke, who devised what he called a "scientific method," which purported to remove the criteria and standards according to which judgments were to be made.[13] Subsequently, an essentially similar approach was rediscovered independently by Beverly Payne,[14] and tested, in its most developed form, in a study of hospital and ambulatory care in Hawaii.[15] The "criteria approach," as this method has come to be called, has since received such wide recognition that is has earned a central position in the projected nationwide system of PSRO's.[16] The sets of criteria that this system will generage will presumably stand as concrete embodiments, if not of quality, at least of acceptable care.

It is this concreteness and specificity that render the "criteria approach" so attractive. It adapts so readily to the computer and the management of mass data. The judgments it yields are likely to be highly replicable. What is at issue is their validity.

In assessing the validity of the "criteria approach," we recognize that we are dealing with a generality. No doubt, the lists of criteria do vary in structure and content and may be put to different uses. For example, the method originally described by Lembcke was applied only to specified surgical operations and used only to judge whether the operation was "justified or criticized," based on the evidence at hand. Even then, the judgment was further tempered by accepting the performance of teaching hospitals as the standard. By analogy, one might expect that the criteria would yield reasonably valid judgments as to the necessity for admission and readiness for discharge, though this is not proven. But do the criteria, as currently designed, represent adequately the quality of care more richly conceived? I shall argue not only that they do not, but also that they most probably *can* not. This means that some of the shortcomings I shall mention can be remedied by better design, but others are so basic that they call for a totally different approach.

All methods of assessment that begin with a sample of hospital records drawn by primary discharge diagnosis or operative procedure share a number of defects. First, the sample excludes all cases that should have been so diagnosed or operated, but were not. Thus, a whole slice of performance remains totally in the dark. Second, there is considerable doubt that performance is so homogeneous that a selection of diagnostic categories that is not a probability sample can stand for the total case load of a physician or an institution.[17] In fact, recent evidence based on a performance index using the criteria approach has shown generally low correlations in the performance of the same physicians across diagnostic categories.[18] Finally, in all instances, the validity of judgments is contingent upon the completeness and accuracy, if not truthfulness, of the material in the record. While it is true that hospital practice and recording are correlated, the level of correlation appears to be low.[19] Even if this correlation were high, the hospital record would ordinarily have little or no information about two important segments of the episode of care: that provided prior and subsequent to hospitalization.

Some additional deficiencies are particularly relevant to the criteria approach as ordinarily designed and implemented. To begin with, no account is taken of the presence of diagnoses additional to the primary one, which may influence management, unless through the assumption that in large samples the presence and influence of such additional diagnoses tends to become comparable. Similarly, no account is taken of redundancy and wastefulness in management, whether in diagnostic investigation or treatment. The emphasis on justification of admission and readiness for discharge is an exception to this general observation. Even here, however, some important deficiencies may intrude. For example, if the criterion is readiness for discharge, without attention to average length of stay, one could lose sight of how long it takes to become fit to leave the hospital, and why. In considering the appropriateness of admission, it is very unusual to raise some questions that should be fundamental to quality assessment: namely, whether the disease could have been prevented in the first place, and whether hospitalization has become necessary, in part, due to prior mismanagement.[20]

Closer to the assessment of hospital care itself, it is very unusual, using the criteria approach, to pass judgment on the accuracy of the discharge diagnosis, the need for surgical intervention, or the choice of operation. These are generally taken as given, and attention is focused on whether the record of prior management includes the minimum set of activities that corresponds to these diagnoses or interventions; no matter what else has been done, how circuitous the path, or how proper the final destination. Strictly speaking, this is a test of internal consistency, which is an attribute at least once removed from quality of performance.

Assuming the discharge diagnosis to be accurate and the minimum criteria set to be relevant, further difficulties arise in constructing an overall measure of performance which requires a summation of component subparts. It is usual to assume equal weights for all the items. Even when, as in the most recent work of Payne, differential weights are assigned, it is not clear on what basis this is done.[21] It is seldom, if ever, recognized that the process of management consists of highly interactive parts and that, when certain key elements are lacking, the care as a whole must be judged to be poor, no matter how many of the other criterion items have been performed and recorded.

CLINICAL JUDGMENT

We have now arrived at what I think is the core of the problem. Clinical management is a complex process of diagnostic and therapeutic decision making. It is based on factual knowledge, but requires something additional, which we recognize as clinical judgment, and which is at the heart and marrow of technical quality. Clinical judgment involves decisions as to what alternatives to consider in diagnosis and therapy; how far to go in seeking what degree of certainty; what means to use; what risks to incur relative to what probability of success in seeking how large a benefit; when to act and when to watchfully wait. What a far cry from the stereotyped behavior embodied in the lists of criteria, which can so easily become an indiscriminate assemblage of the elements of care, so that they are almost a caricature of clinical judgment rather than a true representation. No wonder that physicians are, almost intuitively, repelled by the very thought of being judged by these.

The deficiencies that we have enumerated are not unknown to those who have developed the criteria lists, more recently under the prod of federal programs for quality control. Accordingly, there is much effort to refine what has been pejoratively called the "laundry list" of criteria into something more representative of the realities of the clinical task. This has included the specification of degrees of severity of the major illnesses, and the recognition of frequently encountered combinations of illnesses.[22] A larger forward step is the development of lists that are related to presenting problems, rather than completed diagnoses; and these, in turn, have shaded into what is the opposite pole to the "laundry list": namely, the algorithm and the logic tree. In passing, it is interesting to note that the algorithms which were originally developed to prepare non-physicians to perform clinical tasks, have proved to be so fruitful an approach to the assessment of the clinical skills of the physicians themselves.[23]

The algorithm or the logic tree recognizes that the clinical task begins with a presenting problem, that it proceeds in step-wise fashion, that at each juncture the results of previous steps are taken into account before the next step is taken, and that each step must be justified. Needless to say, the proper progression through this sequence of decisions and activities is prescribed by medical science and by its proper application in the opinion of its leading practitioners. So far, this is the best we can do, but it is by no means the end of the road. The considerations that go into constructing the recommended progression through the logic tree need to be critically examined. No doubt, the decision rules that govern this progression derive from the probabilities of the occurrence of certain states of nature and of the probabilities of risks and benefits attached to alternative courses of action. The validity of these probabilities, which are often subjective, needs to be established. At a more fundamental level of analysis, the recommended content and sequence specified by the logic tree may be considered to constitute a strategy designed to achieve an objective: for example, a diagnosis of specified accuracy and a treatment of specified effectiveness. To this may be added the objective of minimum risk and minimum monetary cost. There may be trade-offs between monetary cost or risk and the degree of uncertainty desired or of the likelihood of error that one is willing to accept. When the strategies devised and adopted are also responsive to social objectives, one has a means of choosing that strategy which promises the most, with the minimum of means, to the largest number of people. Thus, the study of alternative strategies of management, and the choice among them, as dictated by specified objectives, becomes the foundation for both medical education and quality assessment of professional performance.

STYLES AND STRATEGIES

Individual practitioners may differ not only with respect to the strategies they adopt in the management of similar situations, but also with respect to styles, which may be defined as stable and pervasive preferences for certain types of strategies over others. What is problematic is defining what properties of such behavior can be said to constitute categories of style, what constitutes "goodness" in style, and with what justification. With respect to problem solving one might suggest categories such as: stereotypy or routinization versus flexibility, parsimony versus redundancy, degrees of tolerance of uncertainty, variations in the propensity to take risks, and preference for Type I errors versus Type II.[24] With respect to the interpersonal relationship there are equally diverse styles, including the hierarchical versus the egalitarian, and the directive versus the participatory.[25] In the elucidation of these and other properties of styles and strategies we may find much to help us in what is already known about problem-solving and troubleshooting behavior, in general,[26] and about clinical decision making, in particular.[27]

I have not found in the literature of our field studies of styles and strategies that I can describe to you as complete models. But there are some that may indicate the direction of inquiry that I have in mind.

The first study is a review by Howie of what happened to patients who came to the Western Infirmary of Glasgow, Scotland, with signs and symptoms, suggestive of appendicitis.[28] Figure 3 shows an overall accounting of such a cohort. We find that appendectomy was performed in 80 percent of cases. Of these, the majority were found to have an inflamed appendix; but a minority, amounting to 14 percent of the total cohort, had a normal appendix. The removal of normal appendices can, provisionally, be taken to mean that surgery was not justified, and that there has been an error of commission, sometimes referred to as error of Type I. Surgery was not performed

FIGURE 3
Disposition of Patients Admitted With Appendicitis as Initial Diagnosis, by Correctness of Diagnosis (Glasgow, Scotland)

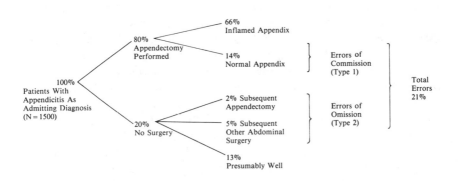

Source: J.G.R. Howie, "The Place of Appendicectomy in the Treatment of Young Adult Patients with Possible Appendicitis, *Lancet*, 1 (June 22, 1968), 1365–1367.

Figure reproduced by permission from *Medical Care Chart Book* (Ann Arbor: School of Public Health, University of Michigan, 1972).

on 20 percent of patients. During the subsequent two years, some of these returned with symptoms which required an appendectomy or some other abdominal surgery, whereas the remainder, amounting to 13 percent of the total cohort, remained well. If one assumes that for those who returned for the subsequent surgery, the earlier decision not to operate had been wrong, one concludes that in 7 percent of the total cohort there was an error of omission, or Type II error. This means that the total error, the sum of Type I and Type II errors, was 21 percent. Thus, this simple accounting procedure reveals an important segment of practice not usually subject to assessment: namely, the consequences of failing to act, or to arrive at a specified diagnosis.

The further investigation of alternative strategies or styles is shown in Figure 4. At the Western Infirmary, there were two groups of surgeons; one more "conservative," or less ready to operate than the other, in the presence of a picture that was suggestive of appendicitis. The top panel in Figure 4 shows the experiences of the two groups. It is clear that the less conservative group, which Howie, perhaps exaggeratedly, calls "radical," performed more appendectomies and, as a result, incurred the removing of more normal appendices; but it also reaped the benefit of a smaller number of patients with recurrent symptoms.

Which of these two strategies, the "conservative" or the "radical," is to be preferred? One answer is provided in the lower part of Figure 4. Given the mortalities from the removal of a normal appendix and the non-removal of a diseased appendix, it is possible to compute the avoidable mortalities for each of the two strategies. This reveals that the less conservative strategy is to be preferred because it yields the lower mortality. Significantly, this conclusion is contrary to the one which would result from considering the frequency of removal of normal tissue, which is the more usual criterion in this situation.

Of course, Howie's conclusion is contingent on the accuracy of his assumptions and his data, both of which can be criticized. It is also restricted to the strategies observed. A still more radical strategy, for example one in which every suspected case were operated, would produce a higher mortality than the "conservative" strategy actually observed. Finally, the framework of evaluation is rather restricted, since it takes account only of mortality, important as that is.

A more inclusive framework for analysis is to be found in a clinical trial of the relative advantages and disadvantages of two methods of treating varicose veins: one by surgery and the other by the injection of sclerosing materials into the veins.[29] The criteria and findings are shown in Table 1. The criteria include not only mortality and morbidity, but also the direct and indirect costs of the two methods of treatment. Fortunately, in this instance, all the criteria favor treatment by injection, provided this is done precisely as described by the trial. Had the findings shown that each method was better in some respects but worse in other respects, we would have needed a method of accounting that could add up morbidity, mortality, and monetary costs into one summary measure. This is a matter to which we have alluded earlier in this paper, and which we have considered in greater detail in another publication.[30]

FIGURE 4
Percent Distribution of Persons (12-29 Years of Age) Admitted for Possible Appendicitis by Whether Operated, Nature of Tissue Removed, and Subsequent Recurrence of Symptoms and by Type of Approach to Surgery (Western Infirmary of Glasgow, Scotland, 1963)

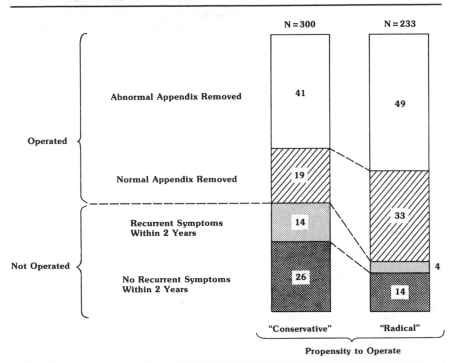

Computation of Expected Avoidable Mortality for Each Approach, Based on Estimates of Risk

State of Appendix	Percent by State	Mortality Risk	Expected Mortality[b]
"Conservative Approach"			
Normal, removed	19	0.02	0.00038%
Abnormal, not removed	8[a]	0.04	0.0032
Both	—	—	0.0070
"Radical Approach"			
Normal, removed	33	0.02	0.0066%
Abnormal, not removed	0	0.04	—
Both	—	—	0.0066

[a] 49% - 41% = 8%
[b] Product of preceding columns

Source: J.G.R. Howie, "The Place of Appendicectomy in the Treatment of Young Adult Patients with Possible Appendicitis, *Lancet,* 1 (June 22, 1968), 1365–1367. Figure reproduced by permission from *Medical Care Chart Book* (Ann Arbor: School of Public Health, University of Michigan, 1972).

TABLE 1

Benefits and Costs of Treating Varicose Veins by Each of Two Methods of Treatment in a Controlled Trial (London, 1967-1968)

	Method of Treatment	
	Injection-Compression Sclerotherapy	Surgery
I. Benefits		
A. At end of 3 years, no further treatment; considered to be improved[a]	86%	78%
II. Costs		
A. Did not attend[b]	6%	15%
B. Mortality risk[c]	1 in 7,000	1 in 4,500
C. Immediate complications[d]	28%	16%
D. Direct monetary costs per case[e]		
1. Capital costs	not estimated	not estimated
2. Current costs		
a. Actual	£ 9.77	£ 44.22
b. Hypothetical[f]		£ 16. or £ 12.
E. Indirect Costs		
1. Mean time for treatment and travel	30 hours	100 hours
2. Mean number of days taken off work	6.4 days	31.3 days
3. Average loss of earnings for those employed full-time	£ 29	£ 118

[a] "There are at present no objective measures of the severity of either symptoms or signs, the limitations of the present methods of assessment are considerable and have to be recognized."

[b] The injection-compression treatment was preferred by 14 out of 18 patients questioned.

[c] Based on a review of the literature.

[d] 28% of those with sclerotherapy developed superficial phlebitis. Of those treated with surgery, 14% developed complications, mainly stitch abscesses and wound infection, and 3% developed neuritis and phlebitis.

[e] Costs refer to 1967-1968 period.

[f] Under assumptions reducing hospital stay and providing treatment in smaller hospitals.

Source: D. Piachaud and J.H. Weddell, "The Economics of Treating Varicose Veins," *International Journal of Epidemiology,* 1 (Autumn 1972), 287-294.

A study that is a better illustration of the concept of strategy in clinical management has been reported recently by Forsyth.[31] The problem is frequent and familiar: how to manage patients who come in with symptoms and findings of pharyngitis so as to achieve greatest success in preventing rheumatic fever at lowest risk and monetary cost. Unfortunately, it is not possible by simple clinical examination to determine accurately whether pharyngitis is caused by the particular type of streptococcus that sometimes triggers subsequent rheumatic fever. To be reasonably certain, at least one throat culture is necessary, which adds to the cost of care and requires some time for the result to be reported. Assuming a diagnosis has been made, penicillin is given either by injection or orally. Penicillin by injection is very effective, but sometimes causes reactions which may be serious enough to be fatal. Oral penicillin is not likely to cause a fatal reaction but is less effective in preventing rheumatic fever, mainly because patients do not adhere to the prescribed regimen. These are the major factors in the situation, at its simplest. They need to be quantified before a choice of strategy can be made.

Table 2 shows the factors and quantities that Forsyth derived from his own experience and from data in the literature. Assuming these to be valid, it is possible to specify the consequences of a course of action, or combinations of such courses, as shown in Table 3. In order to arrive at a summary measure of these consequences, one has to be able and willing, at a minimum (1) to place a money value on the morbidity and loss of life resulting from serious drug reactions and from rheumatic fever, and (2) to account for the monetary cost of the treatment of rheumatic fever as well as the costs of treating the episode of pharyngitis, including the cost of the clinical encounter, of the throat culture, if done, and of the treatment used.[32] Forsyth does not go this far in his analysis. It is notable, however, that monetary cost is a significant factor in his calculation, possibly because he reports from a group practice, where the capitation method of payment is designed to increase the sensitivity of the physician to cost.

TABLE 2
Factors and Quantities Used in the Comparison of Alternative Strategies for the Management of Pharyngitis in Children Without Previous Rheumatic Fever

Distribution of cases of pharyngitis[a]	
Clinically positive	0.359
Clinically questionable	0.184
Clinically negative	0.457
Ratio with positive culture[b]	
Clinically positive	0.536
Clinically questionable	0.279
Clinically negative	0.131
Likelihood of developing rheumatic fever when streptococcal infection is confirmed	
Without treatment	0.005
Penicillin by mouth	0.0003
Penicillin by injection	0.0
Likelihood of fatal reaction	
Penicillin by injection	0.000,0025
Penicillin by mouth	0.0

[a] See the source for the clinical criteria used.

[b] The result of one throat culture is accepted as definitive.

Source: R.A. Forsyth, "Selective Utilization of Clinical Diagnosis in Treatment of Pharyngitis," *Journal of Family Practice* (June 1975), 173–177.

TABLE 3
Consequences of Specified Courses of Action in the Management of Pharyngitis in Children Without Previous Rheumatic Fever, in a Standard Population of 1,000,000 Children

Clinical Diagnosis and Treatment	Number of Cases	Number With Positive Culture	Number With Negative Culture[a]	Number Treated	Rheumatic Fever Among Untreated	Rheumatic Fever Among Treated	Fatal Reactions
Clinically Positive	359,000	192,424	166,576				
Treat none				0	962	—	0.00
Treat all by injection			166,576	359,000	—	0	0.90
Treat all orally			166,576	359,000	—	58	0.00
Culture; treat positives by injection				192,424	0	0	0.48
Culture; treat positives orally				192,424	0	58	0.00
Clinically Questionable	184,000	51,336	132,664				
Treat none				0	257	—	0.00
Treat all by injection			132,664	184,000	—	0	0.46
Treat all orally			132,664	184,000	—	15	0.00
Culture; treat positives by injection				51,336	0	0	0.13
Culture; treat positives orally				51,336	0	15	0.00
Clinically Negative	457,000	59,867	397,133				
Treat none				0	299	—	0.00
Treat all by injection			397,133	457,000	—	0	1.14
Treat all orally			397,133	457,000	—	18	0.00
Culture; treat positives by injection				59,867	0	0	0.15
Culture; treat positives orally				59,867	0	0	0.00

[a] Numbers in rectangles are those treated unnecessarily

Source: Computation made using data in R.A. Forsyth, "Selective Utilization of Clinical Diagnosis in Treatment of Pharyngitis," *Journal of Family Practice* (June 1975), 173–177.

COST CONSEQUENCES

This brings us to the final element in our analysis of the quality of care, which is the contribution of monetary cost to the definition of quality, and the cost consequences of different degrees of quality.

Health professionals, as we all know, are averse to considering monetary cost as an element in the definition of quality. There is the general presumption that everything likely to be beneficial must be done for each patient, irrespective of cost. We have already shown that at the more aggregate levels of analysis, such as the case load or target population, this presumption cannot be sustained, because resources are not limitless, and what we do have must be allocated so that it makes the greatest contribution to the collective good. Even at the individual level, we must recognize that each medical procedure also entails monetary costs to the patient and to his family which curtail their ability to purchase alternative goods and services. At any level of analysis, procedures that give no additional benefits in the information they yield or in their contribution to patient well-being are logically redundant and economically wasteful. Such behavior can only mean that the practitioner is unskilled, thoughtless, or socially irresponsible.

The cost consequences of maintaining a specified level of quality are very complex. More and better care is likely to increase both the direct and the opportunity costs of care. But there are also savings. The elimination of unnecessary care would reduce direct and opportunity costs and eliminate the indirect costs that result from the harmful effects of such care. Good care also yields economic benefits through preventing illness, maintaining higher levels of health, and lengthening productive life. Unfortunately, people who live longer are also likely to develop new diseases which are not susceptible to care and which call for additional costly care.

We know almost nothing about the net result of these contradictory tendencies. We can say, in general terms, however, that the average level of quality that we can buy for a given amount of money can vary greatly. There are ways of getting more for the money. Unfortunately, much of the time, we do not know enough to say what is the best way. It is also true that still further improvements in quality will almost certainly mean more expenditures for care. But, beyond a certain point, further improvements in quality will yield smaller and smaller additional benefits. The cost-benefit relationship is so poorly understood, however, that we are, generally, unable to say at what point additional improvements in quality are simply not worth the additional expense.

Empirical research relative to these questions, which are so fundamental to health care policy, is woefully lacking. A study that stands as a notable exception is an attempt to determine the relationship between the price charged for prescriptions and the quality of pharmaceutical services in a sample of community pharmacies in northern Mississippi.[33] Judgment of quality was based on performance of 13 professional functions in connection with filling test prescriptions and responding to preformulated questions put by trained shoppers. The findings are shown in Figure 5. Each dot in the scatter diagram stands for a pharmacy; and it is clear from the appearance of the scatter that there are wide variations in both quality and price, but that there is no relationship between price and the score of quality. Assuming the judgment of quality to be valid, and the price of the test prescriptions to be representative of all prescriptions, one must wonder what is purchased by the consumer when he pays almost twice as much for comparable quality.

All this has to do with the aggregate cost of quality. There is, in addition, the question of who bears the costs, which is the issue of the incidence of costs. The issue arises most clearly in decisions about the substitution of less costly forms of care for hospital care. Even when the quality of care is not altered by this, the burden of the cost of care may be shifted. This occurs because health insurance excludes some services and covers others unequally. As a result, denying hospitalization, or shortening its duration, may increase out-of-pocket costs to patients, if the substitute services are less fully covered

FIGURE 5

Community Pharmacists by Quality of Professional Performance[a] and by Charge per Prescription (Northern Mississippi, Circa 1973)

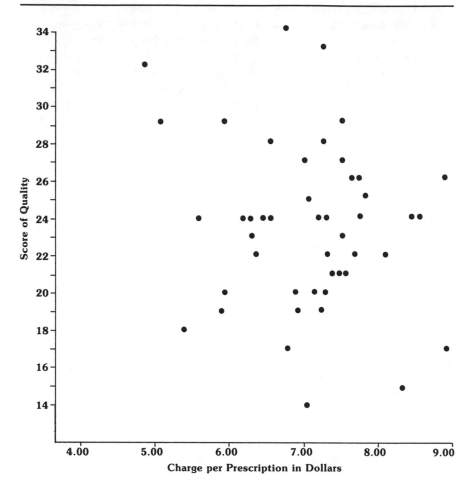

[a] Quality was judged on the basis of performance of 13 professional functions in connection with filling prescriptions for, and responding to pre-formulated questions by, trained "shoppers."

Source: R.A. Jackson and M.C. Smith, "Relations Between Price and Quality in Community Pharmacy," *Medical Care*, 12 (January 1974), 32–39.

or are associated with living expenses, travel, or the like. Thus, savings to the plan may mean added expenditures for the patient, even though he may stand to gain in the long run, due to a slower rise in premiums.

There may be further repercussions. For example, under certain situations, the centralization of care in the hospital may improve physician productivity. Keeping the hospital reasonably full is also efficient for the hospital. This suggests that if the hospital is partially empty, or if it is filled with the most seriously ill, a redistribution will occur, so that the cost of caring for those illnesses that absolutely require hospital care will become significantly higher than it is now, relative to the cost of other care.

None of this should be taken as an argument for careless use of the hospital. It does suggest, however, that the cost consequences of adhering to the criteria of hospital use can be complex: being different in the short run as compared to the long run, and affecting in different ways the plan, the client, the physician, the hospital, the local community, and the nation as a whole.

CONCLUSION

This brings us to the end of our analysis. My purpose in attempting it has not been merely to be critical of the present state of affairs in quality assessment, but to suggest directions for further development. Among these, I believe the following to be particularly useful:

1. Further development of a measure of health status that could represent the final achievement of the health care system.

2. The devising of a battery of proximate, condition-specific outcomes that could be used to monitor and review the conduct of care.

3. Basic research into the process of clinical decision making, so that it can be understood, and ways found to decide what are better ways of achieving specified goals.

4. Research that would result in better understanding of the professional-client relationship and attaching values to specified attributes of it.

5. Understanding the relationship between cost and quality, at the individual and aggregate levels, so that resource allocation decisions can be made rationally.

These and other prospects beckon seductively from the shadows of the future. May good fortune attend us all as we prepare for the journey.

ABOUT THE AUTHOR

At the time of writing, Avedis Donabedian, MD, MPH, was Professor, Department of Medical Care Organization, School of Public Health, University of Michigan, Ann Arbor.

AUTHOR'S NOTE

I have attempted to make this paper a summary of my current thinking and have drawn freely on several previous presentations, with partially overlapping content. These are (1) "A Perspective on Concepts of Health Care Quality," presented at the fall meeting of the Institute of Medicine, November 6, 1974; (2) "Measuring and Evaluating Hospital and Medical Care," presented at the Annual Health Conference of the New York Academy of Medicine, April 24, 1975; (3) "The Quality of Care in a National Health Program," presented before the Subcommittee on Health, of the Committee on Ways and Means, U.S. House of Representatives, July 24, 1975; and (4) "Critical Interfaces in Quality Evaluation," presented at the 27th Institute on Hospital and Community Psychiatry, September 25, 1975.

REFERENCES

1. Mindel C. Sheps, "Approaches to the Quality of Hospital Care," *Public Health Report,* 70 (September 1955), 877–886.

2. A. Donabedian, "Evaluating the Quality of Medical Care," *Milbank Memorial Fund Quarterly,* 44 (July 1966), Part 2, 166–206.

3. Willy De Geyndt, "Five Approaches to Assessing the Quality of Care," *Hospital Administration,* 15 (Winter 1970), 21–42.

4. H.A. Simon, *Administrative Behavior* (New York: Macmillan Co., 1961), 62–66; and O.L. Deniston, I.M. Rosenstock, and V.A. Getting. "Evaluation of Program Effectiveness," *Public Health Reports,* 83 (April 1968) 323–335.

5. Donabedian, "Evaluating the Quality of Medical Care," 194–195, refs. 63–70.

6. The term "outcess" was proposed, also tongue-in-cheek, by Vergil Slee, Director, Commission on Physician and Hospital Activities, Ann Arbor.

7. A further elaboration of this notion is found under the rubric of "health potential" in A. Donabedian, "Models for Organizing the Delivery of Personal Health Services and Criteria for Evaluating Them," *Millbank Memorial Fund Quarterly,* 50 (October 1972), Part 2, 103–154. See, for example, page 107.

8. For one approach to constructing such a measure, see S. Fanshel and J.W. Bush, "A Health Status Index and its Application to Health Service Outcome," *Operations Research,* 18 (November–December 1970), 1021–1060. For an overview of such methods, see R.L. Berg, ed., *Health Status Indexes* (Chicago: Hospital Research and Educational Trust, 1973).

9. Robert L. Hare and Shlomo Barnoon, *Medical Care Appraisal and Quality Assurance in the Office Practice of Internal Medicine* (San Francisco: American Society of Internal Medicine, July 1973). (A more complete report is also available.)

10. H.B. Makover, "The Quality of Medical Care: Methodology of Survey of Medical Groups Associated with the Health Insurance Plan of Greater New York," *American Journal of Public Health,* 41 (July 1951), 825–826.

11. "Mechanism and Purpose," Editorial, *Lancet,* 1 (January 7, 1950), 27–28.

12. J. Ehrlich, M.A. Morehead, and R.E. Trussell, *The Quantity, Quality and Costs of Medical and Hospital Care Secured by a Sample of Teamster Families in the New York Area* (New York: Columbia University, School of Public Health and Administrative Medicine, 1962); and M.A. Morehead, R. Donaldson, et al., *A Study of the Quality of Hospital Care Secured by a Sample of Teamster Family Members in New York City* (New York: Columbia University, School of Public Health and Administrative Medicine, 1964).

13. P.A. Lembcke, "Medical Auditing by Scientific Methods," *Journal of the American Medical Association,* 162 (October 13, 1956), 646–655.

14. B.C. Payne, "Continuing Evolution of a System of Medical Care Appraisal," *Journal of the American Medical Association,* 201 (August 14, 1967), 536–540.

15. B.C. Payne and T.F. Lyons, *Method of Evaluating and Improving Personal Medical Care Quality: Episode of Illness Study* (Ann Arbor: School of Medicine, The University of Michigan, February 1972).

16. *Social Security Amendments of 1972,* P.L. 92–603 (Washington, DC: U.S. Government Printing Office, 1972), "Title XI—General Provisions and Professional Standards Review," 101–117; and M.J. Goran, J.S. Roberts, M. Kellog, J. Fielding, and W. Jessee, *The PSRO Hospital Review System,* supplement to *Medical Care,* 13(4) (April 1975).

17. A. Donabedian, *A Guide to Medical Care Administration. Volume II: Medical Care Appraisal—Quality and Utilization* (New York: American Public Health Association, 1969), "Homogeneity and Heterogeneity," 53–56.

18. T.F. Lyons and B.C. Payne, "Interdiagnosis Relationship of Physician Performance Measures," *Medical Care,* 12 (April 1974), 369–374.

19. L.S. Rosenfeld, "Quality of Medical Care in Hospitals," *American Journal of Public Health,* 47 (July 1957), 856–865; and T.F. Lyons and B.C. Payne, "The Relationship of Physicians' Medical Recording Performance to Their Medical Care Performance," *Medical Care,* 12 (August 1974), 714–720.

20. The aspects of performance mentioned in this sentence were pointed out to me by Paul M. Gertman, Director, Health Services Research and Development Program, Boston University Medical Center.

21. B.C. Payne, ed., *The Quality of Medical Care: Evaluation and Improvement* (Chicago: Hospital Research and Educational Trust, 1976).

22. See, for example, J.S. Gonnella and M.J. Goran, "Quality of Patient Care—A Measurement of Change: The Staging Concept," *Medical Care,* 13 (June 1975), 467–473.

23. For an early example of the use of the logic tree in quality assessment, see O.L. Peterson, E.M. Barsamian, and M. Eden, "A Study of Diagnostic Performance: A Preliminary Report," *Journal of Medical Education,* 41 (August 1966), 797–803.

24. T.J. Scheff, "Preferred Errors in Diagnosis," *Medical Care* (July–September, 1964) 166–172.

25. Thomas S. Szasz and Marc H. Hollender, "A Contribution to the Philosophy of Medicine: The Basic Models of the Doctor-Patient Relationship," *Archives of Internal Medicine,* 79 (May 1956), 585–592.

26. Donabedian, "Evaluating the Quality of Medical Care," 194–195, refs. 63–70.

27. For an early formulation of a probability model of clinical decision making, see R.S. Ledley and L.B. Lusted, "Reasoning Foundations of Medical Diagnosis," *Science,* 130 (July 3, 1959), 9–21. For more recent work, see L.B. Lusted, "Decision-Making Studies in Patient Management," *New England Journal of Medicine,* 284 (February 25, 1971), 416–424; and S. Barnoon and H. Wolfe, *Measuring the Effectiveness of Medical Decisions: An Operations Research Approach* (Springfield, IL: Charles C Thomas, 1972).

28. J.G.R. Howie, "The Place of Appendicectomy in the Treatment of Young Adult Patients with Possible Appendicitis," *Lancet,* 1 (June 22, 1968), 1365–1367.

29. D. Piachaud and J.M. Weddell, "The Economics of Treating Varicose Veins," *International Journal of Epidemiology,* 1 (Autumn 1972) 287–294.

30. A. Donabedian, *Aspects of Medical Care Administration Specifying Requirements for Health Care* (Cambridge, MA: Harvard University Press, 1973), 136–149, 164–179.

31. R.A. Forsyth, "Selective Utilization of Clinical Diagnosis in Treatment of Pharyngitis," *Journal of Family Practice* (June 1975), 173–177.

32. For a brief discussion of this subject see D.P. Rice, "The Economic Value of Human Life," *American Journal of Public Health,* 57 (November 1967), 1954–1966. The methodology is developed in greater detail in D.P. Rice, *Estimating the Cost of Illness,* P.H.S. Pub. No. 947–6 (Washington, DC: U.S. Government Printing Office, May 1966). More recent data are provided in B.S. Cooper and W. Brody, "1972 Lifetime Earnings by Age, Sex, Race and Education Level," *Research and Statistics Note* (Social Security Administration), No. 14 (September 30, 1975).

33. R.A. Jackson and M.C. Smith, "Relations Between Price and Quality in Community Pharmacy," *Medical Care,* 12 (January 1974), 32–39.

The Relationship of Nursing Process and Patient Outcomes

Sue Thomas Hegyvary and
R. K. Dieter Haussmann

Focus on patient outcomes in the assessment of health care services has gained wide acceptance because of the need to document the effectiveness of care. Both the PSRO law and JCAH now require evaluation of the effectiveness of the care provided. Applied to nursing, this focus requires identification of patient outcomes that are influenced by nursing care. Outcome assessment in nursing is complicated by the fact that much of nursing is directed toward psychosocial problems, an area in which there are significant measurement difficulties.

Patient care outcomes can be measured along three broad lines: physical condition, psychological or attitudinal status, and knowledge or learning behavior. Specific criteria for determining outcomes in these areas are now being defined by nurses for a variety of patient populations.[1] The ANA has just concluded a major project to develop methodologies for establishing such criteria.

All of these efforts are proceeding on the assumptions that (1) nursing care affects the outcome of the patient's illness and influences his future health status; and (2) even though nursing shares responsibility for patient care with many health disciplines, there exist identifiable outcomes that are primarily attributable to

Reprinted with permission from *Journal of Nursing Administration,* 6 (November 1976), pp. 18-21, copyright © 1976, J. B. Lippincott Co.

nursing care. Unfortunately, there have been few studies conducted in this area and no data base exists which would allow identification of the consequences of even standard nursing practices. Hegyvary did find that care outcomes of patients undergoing abdominal hysterectomy differed in two hospitals.[2] The data strongly suggested, but did not document in specific terms, that nursing care before and after the operation differed between hospitals. Unfortunately, the lack of inclusion of specific measures of nursing performance (i.e., process) prohibited formulation of conclusions regarding process-outcome relationships. Without understanding this relationship, the meaning and usefulness of patient outcome measures is doubtful.

This study attempted to explore some of the problems involved in addressing the process-outcome relationship for nursing care. It was conducted in the context of a larger study focusing on the development and testing of a process evaluation instrument for nursing care, and is thus only a very limited effort to begin to understand the problems outlined above.[3]

STUDY DESIGN

Considerations in selecting patient populations were: (1) the groups chosen should have illnesses for which specific outcomes could be delineated; (2) the outcomes could be predicted to relate to nursing care; and (3) adequate patient samples would be accessible in two local hospitals in which process monitoring was taking place as part of the larger study. Based on these considerations, patients with congestive heart failure (CHF) and patients undergoing abdominal hysterectomy (AH) were selected.

Patients with CHF were included in the study if they had been in the hospital for at least six days, if they were out of the acute stage of illness, and if they had no known pathological involvement beyond cardiovascular and respiratory systems. Patients were chosen with reference to the American Heart Association Functional Classifications of Patients with Diseases of the Heart.[4] On admission they were class IV, i.e., in an acute stage of illness. They were interviewed six days after admission, when they were generally comfortable and subject only to slight limitations of physical activity, i.e., class II.

The abdominal hysterectomy sample was observed six days postoperatively. Patients were not included in the sample if there was any additional pathological involvement that appeared likely to alter the postoperative course.

These specifications permitted clearer delineation of outcome measures because the degree of pathological involvement was controlled, but they also presented great difficulties in securing an adequate sample within a reasonable period. Particular difficulty was encountered with patients with congestive heart failure. Numerous patients had multiple diseases in addition to the cardiopulmonary illness. The intensity of illness and the anticipated period of resolution of congestive failure are not so clear cut as classification may suggest. Thus, the CHF sample contained only 10 patients, all from the same hospital, and the AH sample numbered 18 patients, 10 from one hospital and 8 from the other, selected over a data collection period of three months.

To test the relationship between nursing process and patient outcomes, it was necessary to develop both process and outcomes instruments for each patient category. A subset of the nursing process criteria that had been developed for the total process evaluation instrument was selected to administer to each type of patient.[5] The criteria were selected to cover the scope of the nursing process and to be of particular relevance to CHF and AH patients, respectively. Thirty-eight criteria were selected for CHF patients, and 24 for patients undergoing abdominal hysterectomy.

Only immediate outcomes of care were measured, as a post-hospitalization study was not feasible. Measurement instruments were based partly on chart audit but also on patient interview and observation. Outcome criteria used are presented in Tables 1-3.

The instruments for measuring physical condition and level of health knowledge had not been previously tested. Thus, content validity is the highest level of validity achieved. The measure of psychological status had been tested previously. It is a modified Affect Adjective Check List developed by Zuckerman, and was used in this study as a card sort for patient's self-report of psychological status.[6]

Data collection was designed to maximize observer reliability. Achieving observer reliability required considerable clarification of each question, specification of the source of information, and clear response categories. Nevertheless, there was still lack of agreement on some items. The health knowledge category presented the greatest problem. Observers often found it difficult to determine what level of patient response comprised an acceptable answer. Information about physical condition derived from written records presented us with a lesser, though troublesome, problem with observer reliability.

The observer reliability problem was handled first by joint observation and interviewing. The three nurses selected for this task went together to the patient care unit, each with the same worksheet. As the record for each patient was reviewed, each observer completed her own worksheet without comparing notes with the others. The three then went to the patient's room, where one nurse conducted the interview while the other two listened. Finally, all responses were compared and points of disagreement were discussed.

This method was successful with the process criteria and with outcome criteria related to physical condition. (The measure of psychological status was not a problem because it was a card sort done by the patient.) Health knowledge measures continued to present some difficulties. The observers were generally aware of items on which there would be disagreement, based on their own difficulty in arriving at the answer. Thus, they decided that, when making the observation alone, they should record the patient's response *verbatim* if they felt the slightest uncertainty about the answer.

TABLE 1
Outcome Assessment Criteria, Congestive Heart Failure Patients

Physical Condition

Items refer to three objectives: (1) maintenance of adequate oxygenation; (2) maintenance of skin integrity; and (3) maintenance of adequate rest and sleep.

Item	Response	
1. Temp. 100.4 or more in past 24 hours.	No	0
	Yes	1
2. Have any episodes of orthopnea been recorded in the past 48 hours? (If #2 was answered "Yes" response, do not ask #3; code 0.)	No	0
	Yes	1
3. If nothing recorded for #2, ask the patient: Is it more difficult for you to breathe when you are lying down than when you are sitting up?	No	0
	Yes	1
4. Is the patient's skin cracked due to dryness? (Observe extremities.)	No	0
	Yes	1
5. Does the patient have any skin lesions, burns or abrasions at pressure points or on the extremities?	No	0
	Yes	1
6. According to the record has the patient become fatigued when performing daily activities in the past 2 days? (If answer was "Yes" to #6, code 0 for #7; do not ask.)	No	0
	Yes	1
7. If nothing has been recorded for #6 ask the patient: Are you able to do your daily activities such as getting dressed, eating or going to the bathroom without getting tired?	No	0
	Yes	1
8. Inability to sleep. (To Patient: For the past 2 nights, have you had difficulty sleeping at least several hours at a time?)	No	0
	Yes	1

Health Knowledge

Items refer to patient's understanding of (1) illness, (2) measures to maintain oxygenation, (3) measures to maintain skin integrity, (4) measures to improve rest and sleep, (5) fluid and nutritional status, and (6) medication.

Item	Response	
1. Can you tell me the name of your illness?	0	Unacceptable
	1	Acceptable
2. How can you change your position in bed to help you breathe more easily?	0	U
	1	A
3. What can you do to relieve congestion in your lungs?	0	U
	1	A
4. What can you do to improve the circulation to your feet?	0	U
	1	A
5. What type of diet are you on?	0	U
	1	A
6. Do you know what types of food, if any, you should not eat because of your condition?	0	U
	1	A
7. What is the reason for restricting any foods?	0	U
	1	A
8. Can you tell me the names of medications you are taking while you are in the hospital?	0	U
	1	A
	Don't know	
	NA	
9. What is the dose? (Digitalis preparation or diuretic, in order of preference)	0	U
	1	A
	Don't know	
	NA	
10. How often will you take this medication?	0	U
	1	A
	Don't know	
	NA	
11. What precautions, if any, should you observe because you take this medication? (Clarify: Are there any special things you should do because you take this medication?)	0	U
	1	A
	Don't know	
	NA	

TABLE 2
Outcome Assessment Criteria, Abdominal Hysterectomy Patients

Physical Condition	Health Knowledge
Items refer to (1) prevention of complications and (2) return of normal gastrointestinal function.	Items refer to understanding of (1) illness and (2) activity, including sexual activity.
Item	**Item**
1. Number of postoperative days temperature was 100.4F or higher.	1. Diagnosis. (To patient: Can you tell me the name of the condition you had that made it necessary for you to have your operation?)
2. Number of the postoperative day on which patient returned to solid diet.	2. Name of the operation. (To patient: Can you tell me the name of the operation you just had?)
3. Total number of postoperative narcotics received.	3. Understanding of operation, in simple terms. (To patient: Would you tell me basically what was done in this operation?)
4. Incidence of complications. (Count 3 points for each complication recorded; e.g., debiscense or abcess, UTI, thrombophlebitis, respiratory congestion, wound infection, etc.)	4. Activity limits after discharge. (To patient: What will your activity limits be when you go home?)
5. Number of days patient was bothered by gas pains. (To patient: Have you been bothered by gas pains since your operation? How many days have you had them?)	5. Effect of operation on sexual activity. (Continued from #4. Do you know if there will be other limitations, such as in sexual relations?)

TABLE 3
Measure of Psychological Status (CHF and AH Patients)

Modified Zuckerman Affect Adjective Check List

Each adjective is typed on a separate card. Patient sorts cards into two stacks: (1) I do feel like this today, and (2) I do not feel like this today. Patient gets one point for each positive word answered positively and each negative word answered negatively. Range of scores is 0 to 19.

Adjective	Affect
1. Angry	−
2. Calm	+
3. Cheerful	+
4. Contented	+
5. Desperate	−
6. Depressed	−
7. Determined	+
8. Frightened	−
9. Happy	+
10. Nervous	−
11. Optimistic	+
12. Panicky	−
13. Secure	+
14. Shaky	−
15. Steady	+
16. Tense	−
17. Terrified	−
18. Upset	−
19. Worrying	−

The question of observer reliability is one of crucial importance that has not been fully addressed in instrument development and testing in the health care evaluation field.

ANALYSIS AND FINDINGS

In the study of the relationship between the nursing process and patient care outcomes, the individual patient was the unit of analysis. The scores for each of the components of the nursing process methodology—Assessing-Planning, Physical Care, Nonphysical Care Evaluation—into which the process criteria were grouped, were correlated with the scores for each outcome category. The results are presented for the two patient groups in Tables 4 and 5.

In the abdominal hysterectomy sample the patient's physical condition correlated with the quality of direct care, both in regard to physical and nonphysical needs. Patient psychological status correlated with the assessing-planning and physical care components; however, contrary to expectation, it was note associated with nonphysical care, which includes psychological-emotional

TABLE 4
Correlation of Nursing Process and Outcomes in Abdominal Hysterectomy

Nursing Process		Patient Outcomes (N = 18)		
		Physical Condition	Psychological Status	Health Knowledge
Assessing—planning	R =	.277	− .36[a]	.145
	P =	.18	.07	.28
Physical care	R =	.484[a]	.395[a]	.144
	P =	.02	.05	.28
Nonphysical care	R =	.517[a]	.049	.310[a]
	P =	.01	.42	.11
Evaluation	R =	− .241	− .206	− .133
	P =	.17	.21	.27

The first figure in each cell is the simple correlation; the second figure indicates level of significance.
[a] Significant at .10 level.

support. The level of health knowledge was correlated with nonphysical care, as predicted, since health teaching is part of that process objective. Most of these findings indicate that the nursing process and patient outcomes were related in a positive direction for this sample.

In the congestive heart failure sample, physical condition was inversely related to the physical care component of the nursing process. In view of the patient sample, this finding appears to indicate that the most severely ill patients were given more attention by the nursing staff. This finding could also indicate that outcomes were not appropriately specified in relation to the severity of illness. Further documentation is required to find a satisfactory explanation.

TABLE 5
Correlation of Nursing Process and Outcomes in Congestive Heart Failure

Nursing Process		Patient Outcomes (N = 10)		
		Physical Condition	Psychological Status	Health Knowledge
Assessing—planning	R =	− .049	− .051	.526[a]
	P =	.44	.44	.05
Physical care	R =	− .463[a]	.101	− .186
	P =	.09	.39	.30
Nonphysical care	R =	.249	.492[a]	.201
	P =	.24	.07	.29
Evaluation	R =	− .055	− .323	.573[a]
	P =	.44	.18	.04

The first figure in each cell is the simple correlation; the second figure indicates level of significance.
[a] Significant at .10 level.

The psychological status of CHF patients was related to the quality of non-physical care, as predicted. However, the level of health knowledge was not related to nonphysical care but to assessment-planning and to evaluation. This finding suggests a possible substitution effect in that assessing, planning, and evaluation require interaction with the patient. Perhaps the nurse's questions for purposes of problem identification and evaluation of the patient's response to therapy added to the health knowledge of the patient.

Although the number of cases was very limited, an attempt was made to determine whether scores differed in relation to the hospital setting. As previously indicated, the AH patients were located in two hospitals. The two hospitals were known to differ along a number of structural dimensions and also to have different overall quality scores. The results showed that Hospital A had significantly lower quality scores in the areas of nonphysical care (psychological-emotional support, health teaching, etc.), and evaluation of care. There was a correspondingly significant difference in the level of health knowledge in the two sets of patients. However, there was no significant difference in psychological status, as was expected in view of the difference in process scores on nonphysical care. The inconsistency in the results suggests that there are probably factors related to the hospital setting that may confound the relationship between the nursing process and patient care outcomes.

CONCLUSION

These findings suggest that the relationship between the nursing process and patient care outcomes is somewhat inconsistent, and may differ with various types of patients. The focus on outcome assessment is supported, as in every type of outcome with both types of patients, some part of the nursing process showed a significant correlation. However, the data suggest that limiting quality assessment to either process or outcome measures may be inappropriate because of the inconsistency of the relationship and the lack of conclusive evidence regarding causes and effects.

ABOUT THE AUTHORS

At the time of writing, Sue Thomas Hegyvary, PhD, RN, was Associate Professor, College of Nursing and College of Health Sciences, Rush University, and Chairperson, Department of Medical Nursing, Rush-Presbyterian-St. Luke's Medical Center, Chicago, Illinois. R. K. Dieter Haussmann, PhD, was Vice President for Research and Development, Medicus Systems Corporation, and Assistant Professor, College of Health Sciences, Rush University, Chicago.

REFERENCES

1. J. W. Taylor, "Measuring the Outcomes of Nursing Care," *Nursing Clinics of North America,* 9(2) (1974), 337-348; M. I. Anderson, "Development of Outcome Criteria for the Patient with Congestive Heart Failure," *Nursing Clinics of North America,* 9(2) (1974), 349-358; and E. Hilger, "Developing Nursing Outcome Criteria," *Nursing Clinics of North America,* 9(2) (1974), 323-330.

2. S. T. Hegyvary, "Organizational Setting and Patient Care Outcomes: An Exploratory Study," doctoral dissertation, Vanderbilt University, 1974.

3. R. K. Dieter Haussmann, et al., *Monitoring Quality of Nursing Care, Part II: Assessment and Study of Correlates,* DHEW Pub. No. HRA 76-7 (Washington, DC: U.S. Department of Health, Education & Welfare, July 1975).

4. Anderson, "Development of Outcome Criteria for the Patient with Congestive Heart Failure."

5. The instrument is described in S. T. Hegyvary and R. K. Dieter Haussmann, "Monitoring Nursing Care Quality," *Journal of Nursing Administration,* 6 (November 1976), 3-12.

6. M. Zuckerman, "The Development of an Affect Adjective Check List for the Measurement of Anxiety," *Journal of Consulting Psychology,* 24 (1960), 457-461.

Criterion Measures of Nursing Care Quality

Barbara J. Horn and Mary Ann Swain

INTRODUCTION

This study addresses the issue of evaluating the quality of nursing care provided adult, medical-surgical, hospitalized patients. The increasing complexity of health care, changing societal demands for services, and the thrust to provide quality care to more people in a more efficient and more accessible manner, necessitates systematic objective evaluation of the delivery of health care services. Nursing constitutes the largest number of health professionals functioning in acute-care facilities and nurses are responsible for the patient continuously from admission to discharge. The impact of nursing care services must be measured.

Existing evaluation tools in nursing reflect measures of structure and process. Little research effort has been devoted to the development and testing

Reprinted from *Criterion Measures of Nursing Care Quality,* National Center for Health Services Research, Research Summary Series, DHEW Pub. No. (PHS) 78-3187 (Hyattsville, MD: Public Health Service, U.S. Department of Health, Education & Welfare, August 1978). The complete report of this research is found in B. J. Horn and M. A. Swain, *Development of Criterion Measures of Nursing Care,* Vol. I, *Reliability Test Results and Instrument of Health Status Measures;* Vol. II, *Manual for Instrument of Health Status Measures* (Springfield, VA: National Technical Information Service, 1976).
The research described in this article was performed under NCHSR grant HS 01649.

of outcome measures. It is recognized that patient outcomes arise from multiple determinations. Outcomes are the combined result of several converging forces: the restorative process inherent within each individual, environment, and social influences, and the contributions of all participative health professionals (i.e., nurses, physicians, physical therapists, social workers). Nevertheless, a method to assess nursing's impact on patients' health status is urgently needed.

The objective of the project was to develop, refine, and validate measures of the quality of nursing care. The focus was on the assessment of the outcomes of the nursing care process as reflected by the patients' health status. Measures of patients' physical and emotional status, and the extent of their knowledge and ability to perform self-care, were developed and related to universal and health deviation demands. Thereafter, the investigators sought to ascertain the reliability and validity of each of the various measurement items generated. Due to the research and developmental focus of the work, no specific hypotheses were formulated or tested. A total of 539 measurement items were developed and validated, using eight universal and 10 health deviation self-care demand categories developed by Orem.[1] In addition, 414 of the items were pretested to determine deviations in findings returned by different observers. This subjective variation was corrected by the development of specific observation procedures for specific patient groups. The validated measurement items and an "instrument" for matching observer techniques to particular patients were incorporated in a manual.[2]

Analytical and Methodological Procedures

A comprehensive instrument for measuring the quality of nursing care depends on specifying the domain of care for which nursing is responsible. A major difficulty from the beginning was that nursing did not have a well-defined classification system for identifiable patient care problems. Thus, it was necessary to adopt at least a rudimentary system for organizing and defining nursing care problems. Three approaches were explored; a discussion of each approach follows.

Initially, specific medical diagnoses were chosen as a heuristic device to structure our thinking about nursing care problems. Frequently, occurring medical diagnoses were identified for medical-surgical hospitalized patients. Sources included Payne, the Commission of Professional and Hospital Activities (CPHA), and the National Center for Health Statistics (NCHS).[3] For each medical diagnosis nursing care problems were identified, the ameliorative activities for each problem were listed, and the desired outcomes for those activities were described. Finally, those desired outcomes were translated into quantifiable measures, usually subsets of questions to ask or observations to make about patients.

It soon became obvious that the disease entity classification was too detailed and repetitious to be appropriate for nursing. That is, patients classified differently by medical diagnoses were often similar in terms of nursing problems. For example, the paraplegic rehabilitation patient and the major stroke patient who is scheduled for prolonged bedrest are both at risk in terms of skin breakdown. Respiratory criteria for patients following surgery with a general anesthetic are appropriate measures of effective nursing care whether the operation was a herniorrhaphy, cholecystectomy, hysterectomy, or a total hip repair. In each case, the criteria assess the effectiveness of deep breathing and coughing exercises.

Our second approach was to define nursing problems by focusing on the various systems of the body, e.g., respiratory, renal, and cardiovascular. Continued testing of the instrument and development of the measurement item revealed the limited usefulness of this approach. For example, within a systemic class such as "gastrointestinal," whether the patient is hospitalized for cholelithiasis which requires surgical intervention or for medical therapy alone makes considerable difference with respect to the nursing problems presented by that patient. Furthermore, it was our experience that when nurses focused on a single system they tended to ignore relevant outcomes that involved other systems. For example, outcomes related to problems of elimination were missed for patients with cardiovascular conditions. Systemic classifications do not define mutually exclusive and exhaustive classes of patients which reflect unique sets of nursing care problems.

A third alternative, which avoids these problems, focuses on the bio-psycho-social functioning of individuals rather than on systemic problems or disease entities. Areas of healthy functioning of considerable interest to nursing include the patient's ability to take in air, food, and water; to distribute these necessities for life throughout the body; and to carry away the waste products of their utilization. In addition to general physical health, nurses are interested in those health behaviors that afford the individual a productive, meaningful life. Nurses are concerned about the person's ability to work, rest, think, play, and love.

An organizing framework defining more carefully these outcomes has been derived from earlier work by Dorothea Orem. This model is based upon the premise that the special concern of nursing is, "man's need for self-care action and the provision and management of it on a continuous basis in order to sustain life and health, recover from disease or injury, and cope with their effects."[4] Self-care, the ability to do activities of normal living, consists of two kinds, universal and health deviation. Universal self-care includes all demands necessary for activities of daily living. Health deviation self-care demands arise in the events of illness, injury or disease. For evaluating nursing care, the patient's health status was measured along dimensions related to these requirements for self-care.

Nine categories of health status dimensions were developed from Orem's description of self-care requirements related to air; water/fluid intake; food; elimination of body wastes; rest/activity/sleep; solitude, social interaction and productive work; protection from hazards; normality; and health deviation. These nine aspects of health provided the necessary framework for organizing nursing care outcomes. For further specificity in defining the domain of nursing care, each of the categories of health status was subdivided into four areas: (I) Evidence that the requirement is met; (II) Evidence that the person has the necessary knowledge to meet the requirement; (III) Evidence that the person has the necessary skills and performance abilities to meet the requirement; and (IV) Evidence that the person has the necessary motivation to meet the requirement.

This nine-by-four framework for describing the scope of nursing's responsibility was a valuable heuristic device for the generation of patient outcome variables. The nurse staff selected seven of the nine categories for initial focus (air, water, food, elimination, rest/activity/sleep, normality of skin, and health deviation) and proceeded to list all the variables indicated by the domains I-IV for each category. For example, variables were generated that would demonstrate the degree to which the patient's universal demand for air has been met (domain I), the adequacy of knowledge necessary to meet his/her need for air following hospitalization (domain II), and his/her ability and motivation to effectively manage self-care related to getting air (domains III and IV). Normal or optimum levels of achievement were also described for each variable generated. In the health deviation category, ten subsets of dimensions associated with health deviation and related therapies were generated (IV and wound observations, knowledge of health deviation, medication knowledge and injection performance, knowledge of diet, fluids, exercises, activity restrictions, recommended rest, special appliances, and skin-wound care) (see Table 1).

Validation Procedures

Two criteria for content validity have been proposed by Nunnally and Durham.[5] These criteria are that the measures should be representative of the domain to be covered, and that the design of the measures should use "sensible methods" of construction. In order to establish content validity, three groups reviewed the variables and advised on the completeness and appropriateness of their content with regard to nursing. These groups also advised on the reasonableness of suggested measurement techniques.

First, the lists of variables generated for each of the areas of health status were reviewed by all members of the research staff. Specific variables were judged as appropriate or inappropriate by collective opinion as to whether or not a particular variable was a reflection of nursing activities. Lists of appropriate variables were submitted to the National Advisory Panel, and

TABLE 1
Number of Measurement Items in Health Status Categories and Domains

Categories	Total Measurement Items in Domains				
	I Requirements Met	II Knowledge	III Performance	IV Motivation	Total
Universal Dimensions					
1. Air	41	6	20	3	70
2. Water	19	5	5		29
3. Food	3	3	16		22
4. Elimination	16	16	41		73
5. Rest/activity/sleep	67		43		110
6. Solitude and social interaction	1				1
7. Protection from hazards					
8. Normality	23				23
Subtotal	170	30	125	3	328
Health Deviation Dimensions					
9. Health deviation I: IV and wound observation	28				28
10. Health deviation II		13			13
11. Medications		31	30		61
12. Therapeutic diet		23	(Injections)		23
13. Therapeutic fluids		11			11
14. Recommended exercises		17			17
15. Physical activity restrictions		11			11
16. Recommended rest		13			13
17. Special appliances		15			15
18. Skin-wound care		19			19
Subtotal	28	153	30	3	211
Total	198	183	155	3	539

evaluated by the following two criteria: (1) the relative completeness of the listings, and (2) the degree to which each variable could be considered an index of the efficacy of nursing activities. Once variables were evaluated in this manner, the National Advisory Panel was asked to rank the variables, using professional judgment, and to weight the relative appropriatenesss of the variable as an index of nursing care, to advise on the possibilities of devising meaurements for the variable, and to determine the significance of a healthy outcome for patients with respect to that particular variable. Following the meeting with the Advisory Panel, variable lists were revised. The third step in establishing content validity for each variable was to ask clinical nurse specialists practicing in acute care settings to evaluate the completeness of each of the variable lists, to judge the appropriateness of each variable as an index of nursing care, and to rank the variables using the same criteria as those employed by the Advisory Panel. The final lists of revised variables and their rankings are listed in the Manual for each category.[6]

Measurement techniques were then sought or developed by project staff for only those variables which were valued as having content validity and a high to moderate sensitivity to nursing care quality. Almost all of these variables fell within domains I-III. (See Table 1 for the numbers of measurement items in each category and domain.) These measurement techniques compose current instrument. Data collection was designed to use the patient as the primary source of data, so direct physical observations and interviews are the most common types of measurement techniques developed. The measures were designed so the staff nurses could readily be trained to do the observations-interviews, and so that the equipment required would be available in most hospitals or could be obtained without great expense.

The remaining three categories of health status variables (solitude and social interaction, protection from hazards, and the remainder of normality) were generated as well, and initial evaluation of their validity was begun with clinical nurse specialists. Many of these variables are concerned with measurement of emotional or affective states. Valid and reliable measurement techniques for affective variables, such as the Gottschalk Clinical Rating Scale of Anxiety and the Word Adjective Checklist, have been documented in the psychology and social psychology literature. These techniques are appropriate for hospitalized patients who experience difficult adjustments to their health problems. Such measurement techniques can be incorporated into the existing instrument.[7]

INTEROBSERVER RELIABILITY PROCEDURES

Nurse staff members were used to establish interobserver reliability for each measurement item. Pairs of nurse staff members were randomly assigned to measure appropriate items for selected patients. A single reliability trial consisted of a pair of observers who approached a patient jointly. One randomly chosen member of the pair directed the interview and performed the tests indicated while the other member observed. For physical examination items, each observer performed the necessary observations and recorded the results. In all trials both observers recorded their observations and scored patient responses independently. These records were returned to a third party who compared the records and reported the results of each trial for each variable as an instance of agreement or disagreement.

The criteria for determining that the measurement technique for a particular variable was invariant over observers were: (1) a sample reliability index of at least 0.80; (2) an alpha error of 0.05; and (3) the lower bound of the 95 percent confidence interval to exclude the reliability index of 0.60.

Decisions on Variables That Fall Below the Standard

A general model for decision-making on the nature of subsequent work required when a reliability test for a variable failed appears in Figure 1. Essentially, the project staff would review the data on a variable to determine if there was a correct method of measuring the variable. If so, information from individual observers was reviewed to determine which persons may have measured variables incorrectly. It appeared reasonable to question the adequacy of the training of observers as the first possible source of unreliability. First remedies for unreliability were to reopen discussions on particular measures to retrain the observers.

When it was shown that training was not the problem, test results that failed to show interobserver reliability argued strongly for the necessity of revising the measuring technique for a particular variable. The last node of the decision-tree then became important. Given the principle that one never has resources sufficient to accomplish all tasks to be done, we sought to maximize the utility of the total instrument by working first on those variables that described outcomes for the greatest number of patients. We decided to work only on those variables that were appropriate for at least 20 percent of the patients covered by the instrument. The remainder of the project's resources went into conducting the reliability and validity tests of those other variables. Variables that failed the reliability test and did not meet the applicability criterion stated above were set aside.

SCOPE OF THE CURRENT INSTRUMENT

Validation procedures utilizing the project staff, the National Advisory Panel and the clinical nurse specialists have resulted in an instrument containing 539 measurement items. Of these measurements, 328 are related to the universal demands, for air (70), food (22), elimination (73), water (29), rest/activity/sleep (110), solitude and social interaction (1), and normality (23). The health deviation section of the instrument (211 measurements) describes intravenous and wound observations (28), patients' knowledge and self-care abilities relative to their health problems (13), their medications (61), therapeutic diet (23), and fluid intake (11), prescribed rehabilitative exercises (17), restrictions on physical activity (11), skin and wound care (19), the use of special appliances (15) and recommended rest (13).[8]

Domains I-III are quite evenly represented over the instrument. There are 198 variables in Domain I (Universal, 170 variables; Health Deviation, 28 variables). Domain II is represented by 183 variables (30 in Universal categories, 153 in Health Deviation). Domain III includes 155 variables (Universal, 125; Health Deviation, 30). Domain IV, which requires affective measures, currently has 3 variables (see Table 1).

FIGURE 1
Decision Tree for Action Following Failure of Reliability Test for a Variable

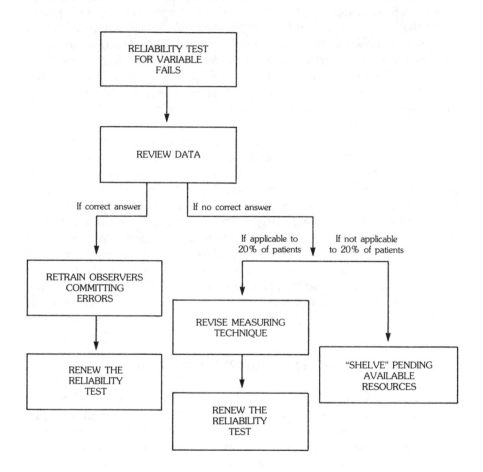

Table 2 gives an overview of the types of items in the instrument. Of the instrument items, 469 are appropriate as quality measures: 414 of these were tested for reliability; the other 55 items were revised or developed after testing was completed and therefore require further tests. The remaining 70 informational items aid interpretation of the quality measures and do not require reliability tests.

Finally, we have drafted health status dimensions and levels of achievement, but not meaurement techniques, in the areas of solitude-social interaction, protection from hazards, and a large portion of normality. Future research is planned to search out appropriate measures in the literature for these health status dimensions.

TABLE 2
Type and Status of Measurement Items in Current Instrument

Component	Quality Measurement Items			Informational Items (reliability tests unnecessary)	Total Items
	Tested for Reliability	Revisions or New Items	Total		
Universal					
1. Air	65	2	67	3	70
2. Water	25	2	27	2	29
3. Food	15	4	19	3	22
4. Elimination	44	1	45	28	73
5. Rest/activity/sleep	83	4	87	23	110
6. Solitude and social interaction	1		1		1
7. Protection from hazards					
8. Normality	18	5	23		23
Health Deviation					
9. Health deviation I: IV and wound observation	23	5	28		28
10. Health deviation II	12	1	13		13
11. Medications	46	12	58	3	61
12. Therapeutic diet	20	2	22	1	23
13. Therapeutic fluids	7	1	8	3	11
14. Recommended exercises	13	3	16	1	17
15. Physical activity restrictions	6	4	10	1	11
16. Recommended rest	10	2	12	1	13
17. Special appliances	11	4	15		15
18. Skin-wound care	15	3	18	1	19
Total	414	55	469	70	539
Percent of total items	77%	10%	87%	13%	

VALIDITY

Content validity has been established for all 539 measurements on the basis of two criteria: that the items in the instrument be representative of the domain to be covered by that instrument, and that the design of the measures themselves utilize "sensible methods" of construction.[9] Variables identified within the instrument were chosen because they represented physiological, psychomotor, cognitive, or affective components of each of the areas of concern to nursing, whether related to universal demands or to demands arising from health deviation. Opinions of the quality staff about the representativeness of each variable as an indicant of the quality of nursing care were verified by two additional groups of experts, the practicing clinical specialists and the National Advisory Panel. The "reasonableness" of suggested measuring techniques was also subjected to critical confirmation by the two groups.

Validation – Case Examples

As reliability testing was being done, anecdotal notes about the process were recorded and cases of special interest were described. Several cases demonstrate some degree of construct validity for several of the measures.

Two such measures were in the component "air." The performance test for the health status dimension "adaptation to activity" is a measure of the patient's ability to adjust his performance of activities of daily living to his needs for oxygen. The variables measured are degrees of shortness of breath, recovery heart rates, and recovery respiratory rates. If the patient is satisfactorily adjusting his activity to his needs, his heart and respiratory rates should return to resting levels within 90 seconds after completing the activity. Most patients tested for this item had respiratory disease causing shortness of breath on exertion. Most of the patients achieved the normal recovery levels within 90 seconds, taking as many rest stops as they needed. In one case, however, a patient, who had congestive heart failure and asthma, did not rest as needed, but in fact hurried through her assigned activity, bathing at the bedside, in order to get ready for some visitors. She notably failed to meet the recovery levels at the 90-second limit. For this patient, the measures were indeed sensitive to the patient's adjustment of her activity levels.

A second measure in the "air" component deals with the patient's emotional adjustment to chronic cough and sputum production. The questions focus on the patient's solutions to any embarrassment or value conflict caused by coughing and expectoration. Overall, responses indicated that the respiratory disease patients interviewed had either adjusted to the point that they felt no embarrassment or had developed adequate solutions. In one case, however, the patient, who had restrictive lung disease and bronchitis, expressed solutions that included extensive withdrawal from social contacts and outside activities. She viewed these solutions as the only course open; yet her expression of frustration and anger indicated her lack of satisfaction with these solutions. Thus the questions have been found to elicit both positive and negative feeling states related to adaptation to a disease process.

Several cases demonstrate construct validity for performance measures in the "food" component. The measures test the patient's avility to perform activities of eating, such as mashing, cutting food, pouring and lifting and opening containers. For a patient with a 17-year history of rheumatoid arthritis, the measures demonstrated inability to mash food and some difficulty in cutting. The patient was suffering a "flare-up" of his arthritis and stated that he usually could manage these activities at home. When asked for his opinion as to whether the tests would demonstrate at discharge any problems he would have at home, he stated "yes, it certainly would." For another patient, with a diagnosis of multiple sclerosis, the measures demonstrated that the muscle weakness in his hands and arms, which had prevented him from lifting a quart container of liquid at home, had resolved to the extent that he could lift it at the time of discharge. He, too, stated that these tests were appropriate for evaluating his abilities to eat at home.

The observers have also noted that the range of motion, muscle strength, muscle endurance, and coordination measures in the Rest/Activity/Sleep component have distingusihed problems with motion from those of strength, and/or coordination. The rheumatoid arthritic's coordination and strength tests were fairly normal depite a notably decreased range of motion. This was the same patient who had difficulty mashing and cutting food. Thus the tests indicated that it was primarily his more limited range of motion which was affecting his eating activity. Another patient demonstrated good strength on the muscle strength-endurance tests except in his hands and feet. The range of motion tests also showed some minor restrictions in hands and feet. After the interview, the patient told the observers that he did have some restricted motion in his hands and feet due to a past history of myasthenia gravis, information that was not pertinent to his present diagnosis and did not appear on the face sheet of the patient record. The loss of motion and strength was not large enough to significantly affect his daily activities. Thus the measures were sensitive to a relatively minor loss of function. Strength and active-passive range of motion tests corroborated, suggesting that the loss of strength had apparently allowed some minor contractures to develop.

Because all of these observations were done for purposes of establishing reliability, the measures were not necessarily obtained at the times most appropriate for evaluation of nursing care. They do, however, demonstrate that the measures are sensitive to differences in patients' health status. If obtained at appropriate times, the tests could validly indicate (for groups of similar patients) strengths and deficiences in the care; that is, whether nurses followed procedures to prevent contractures and to maintain muscle strength, adequately prepared patients for performing daily activities at home, or assisted patients to resolve problems related to adjustment to disease.

RELIABILITY

Of the 414 quality measures in the instrument (see Table 2), 109 or 26 percent attained the stringent criteria set for reliability. That is, for those 109 measures the pairs of nurse observers showed a 0.80 index of agreement which was statistically significant at the 0.05 level; further, the confidence limits for that coefficient excluded the 0.60 index at its lower bound. An additional 31 measures were shown to meet at least two of the criteria; the index of agreement was 0.80 or better and was statistically significant at the 0.05 level. The criterion with respect to confidence bounds was not attained for 140 measures because agreement was absolute ($r = 1.00$) and, thus, no bounds were determinable. These 280 measures which have shown reliability cut across the scope of the instrument. For most sections of the instrument, at least some of the measures are both valid and reliable. The summary of these findings are tabulated in Table 3.[10]

One hundred and eight of the measures need further testing because interobserver reliability was not established for these measures. Another problem arose for the remaining 26 measures. These particular measures appear to be appropriate only for a limited subset of the population, hospitalized adult patients. We were unable to find sufficient persons for whom such measures could be used, despite persistent attempts. These measures would appear to have limited utility for assessment of the quality of nursing care, since few patients would be available to determine an index of quality.

MANUAL

In order for others to utilize the items appropriately and to measure each item reliably, it was necessary to prepare a manual with detailed instructions on the use of the instrument.

The manual supplies information about the patient observations, interviews, scoring procedures, and other guidelines for recording accurate information about the health status of a particular patient.[11] It also includes guidelines for deciding whether or not a particular measurement item is appropriate for patients in various diagnostic categories. The manual is intended to be useful both for training of nurse observers and also as a reference source during actual data collection periods. An overview of its development is described below.

Development of Manual

As each measurement technique was designed, instructions to the observer/interviewer on how to perform the measure were developed. To aid evaluation of the observations and responses, norms or standards documented

TABLE 3
Summary of Reliability Testing on the Instrument

	Number of Measurement Items Meeting Criteria					
Component	Index = .80 a <.05 Lower bound <.60	Index = .80 a <.05	Index = 1.00	Index <.80	Insuf- ficient Patients	Total
Universal						
1. Air	33	6	11	15		65
2. Water	8	1	12	3	1	25
3. Food	2	1	9	3		15
4. Elimination	7		29	8		44
5. Rest/activity/sleep	13	9	32	29		83
6. Solitude and social interaction			1			1
7. Protection from hazards						
8. Normality	11		4	3		18
Health Deviation						
9. Health deviation I: IV and wound observation	13	5	5			23
10. Health deviation II	3	2		7		12
11. Medications	11	2	16	17		46
12. Therapeutic diet	2	2	2	13	1	20
13. Therapeutic fluids		1	2	3	1	7
14. Recommended exercises					13	13
15. Physical activity restrictions			2	4		6
16. Recommended rest					10	10
17. Special appliances	6		4	1		11
18. Skin-wound care		2	11	2		15
Total items	109	31	140	108	26	414
Percent of tested items	26%	8% Reliable 280 (68%)	34%	26%	6% Not reliable 134 (32%)	

in the literature were incorporated into the manual. In those cases where documented "correct" responses were not available, examples of acceptable responses were listed. Three sections of the manual have fairly extensive lists of "correct" responses: Health Deviation Knowledge, Medications, and Special Appliances. For Health Deviation Knowledge, correct responses were detailed for H-ICDA diagnostic categories frequently occurring in several hospitals of varying size, character, and location. For the Special Appliances and Medication components, correct response lists were prepared for commonly prescribed medications and appliances.

After reliability testing was completed, the manual was revised and improved, incorporating knowledge gained from the use of the instrument in data collection. It currently includes an introduction to the instrument and its use; instructions to data collectors; guidelines for reliability testing; equipment needed; detailed descriptions of each instrument component, including the complete lists of health status dimensions generated; a guide for selection and matching of patients and appropriate measures; a discussion of interviewing techniques; and procedures for scoring responses.

Patient Selection Guide

The patient selection guide (Appendix B of the Manual) designates the appropriate health status dimensions to measure for 90 frequently occuring H-ICDA diagnostic categories. It was generated with extensive input by clinical nurse specialists in order to determine which items would be appropriate measures of nursing care for specific patient groups. It was used extensively during reliability testing and is viewed as a substantial beginning effort to match measures to patients in a valid way to evaluate quality of nursing care. By linking H-ICDA code categories to appropriate sets of measurement items in the instrument, the matrix capitalizes on the information system already available in hospital settings. The guide can be used in various geographical locations and is amenable to computerization. It is feasible that both patient selection and production of appropriate data collection materials could be computerized as linked operations using this matrix.

SUMMARY

The work of the project staff has yielded an instrument for measuring patients' health status along a number of dimensions under the influence of nursing care. The project staff considers all measures where the sample interobserver reliability index was at least 0.80 (a < .05) to be reliable. Failure to achieve the confidence limit criterion was a matter of insufficient trials to stabilize the reliability index above the 0.60 lower confidence bound. Therefore, we posit an instrument of 348 valid and reliable measures for general use in assessing the quality of nursing care based on observations of patients' health status. These measures include 280 reliable quality measures and 68 informational data items (see Table 3). For the universal categories they total 248 items, and include air (53), water (23), food (15), elimination (64), rest/activity/sleep (77), solitude and social interaction (1) and normality (15). The remainder of the instrument (100 measures) relates to demands arising from health deviations. Included in this section of the instrument are observations of IV sites and wounds (23), measures of health deviation knowledge (5), medication knowledge (18), injection performance (14), therapeutic diet knowledge (7), knowledge of therapeutic fluids (6), knowledge of physical activity restrictions (3), use of special appliances (10), and care of the skin and wounds (4).

The measures focus on the patient as the primary source of data, and thus require skills in physical observation and interviewing techniques. This necessitates selecting or training appropriately skilled nurse-observers. Needed equipment is readily available and inexpensive.

The instrument as designed is most appropriate for research on alternative models for the delivery of nursing care services. Subsections of the instrument may be used to assess the relative efficacy of alternative nursing care interventions for particular patient problems. Selected items could be used in quality assurance programs at the discretion of the users. For any of these applications, a manual accompanies the instrument in order that others may use each of the measures reliably and effectively.

ABOUT THE AUTHORS

At the time of writing, Barbara J. Horn, PhD, RN, and Mary Ann Swain, PhD, were at the Department of Hospital Administration, School of Public Health, University of Michigan, Ann Arbor.

REFERENCES

1. Dorothea E. Orem, *Nursing: Concepts of Practice* (New York: McGraw-Hill, 1971).

2. B. J. Horn, and M. A. Swain, *Development of Criterion Measures of Nursing Care,* final report to the National Center for Health Services Research, Vol. II, *Manual for Instrument of Health Status Measures* (Springfield, VA: National Technical Information Service, 1976).

3. B. Payne, ed., *Hospital Utilization Review Manual* (Ann Arbor: University of Michigan Medical School, Department of Postgraduate Medicine, 1968); Commission on Professional and Hospital Activities, *Length of Stay in PAS Hospitals, United States, 1971* (Ann Arbor: University of Michigan Press, 1972); and National Center for Health Statistics, *Inpatient Utilization of Short-Stay Hospitals by Diagnoses, United States—1971,* Pub. No. (HRA) 75–1767 (Washington, DC: U.S. Department of Health, Education & Welfare, July 1974).

4. Orem, *Nursing: Concepts of Practice.*

5. J. C. Nunnally and R. C. Durham, "Validity, Reliability, and Special Problems of Measurement in Evaluation Research," in E. L. Strueming and M. Guttentag, eds., *Handbook of Evaluation Research* (Beverly Hills, CA: Sage, 1975), 289–352.

6. Horn and Swain, *Manual for Instrument of Health Status Measures,* Appendix III.

7. See ibid., Appendix III.

8. See ibid., Appendix II, for the instrument.

9. Nunnally and Durham, "Validity, Reliability, and Special Problems of Measurement in Evaluation Research."

10. Findings for the total item set are tabulated in Horn and Swain, *Manual for Instrument of Health Status Measures,* Appendix I, Reliability Test Measures.

11. Ibid., Appendix III.

Status of Quality Assurance in Public Health Nursing

Charlotte Januska, Jane Engle, and Jean Wood

This paper was based on a survey of public health nursing institutions conducted in 1975 by the Quality in Nursing Care Committee of the Public Health Nursing Section of the American Public Health Association. The committee's task was to identify, review, and promote systematic study of issues and factors that influence the provision of high-quality care by public health nurses. Originally presented at the 1976 annual meeting of the American Public Health Association, it is reprinted here for the first time in published form, slightly edited due to space considerations.

INTRODUCTION

While evaluation of care provided is one of the basic steps of the nursing process, the transformation of this step into a quality assurance program in public health nursing is arduous and often elusive. The diversity of services and differing organizational, social and political structures make the operationalization of quality complex in public health nursing. While funding sources often require quality controls, less attention has been focused on the assessment and

Reprinted with permission from a paper presented to the Annual Meeting of the American Public Health Association, Public Health Nursing Section, December 1976.

assurance of quality in community than in hospital settings. Reasons include low priority and visibility of ambulatory, preventive, and home care and methodological difficulties from cumbersome records, problem classification and client characteristics.

Despite these difficulties, there has never been a lack of perceived or real need for quality of care evaluation in public health nursing. This need involves a series of evaluations from individual provider to agency level. Evaluation at the individual level includes an assessment of the progress and effectiveness of care to any given patient or family. Caseloads must be evaluated for appropriateness of selection, casefinding efforts and aggregate patient progress. Selected types of interventions and equipment must be assessed for relation benefit and costs. All aging personnel must be evaluated periodically for continued employment and promotion. Agencies must assess the existence of the needs in the community that can be influenced by public health nursing, the impact of program and the cost-effectiveness of services. Evaluation of all these segments and levels cannot be deferred to some other time or to some other person.

The health care literature contains many articles and reports on quality assurance, however, only a small percent of these are directly and practically applicable to public health nursing. Since 1960, several reports were published that formed the basis of quality related public health nursing research. The thrust of most of this literature was on structure and/or process with a few methods offering the beginnings of outcome study. Among the most well known are Freeman and Lowe's family coping estimate, in which the nurse rates coping ability in nine categories which can be considered independent of a medical or developmental diagnosis,[1] and Mickey's method of identifying extra hospital nursing needs, in which clients are interviewed about 18 categories of public health concerns with nursing needs and family coping ability determined subsequently by the nurse.[2]

Roberts and Hudson presented a method to study patient progress based on the nurse's listing of needs developed while planning care and assessment of changes in needs over time.[3] Highwriter studied characteristics of nurses associated with a reduction of health needs of families receiving public health nursing service.[4] Johnson and Hardin conducted an exploratory study on the content and dynamics of home visits by public health nurses in which the character of selected interactional dimensions were described and factors and forces associated with variations in patient and nurse behavior identified.[5] Holliday published a descriptive study of public health nurses with care to non-well population responsibilities, and focused on utilization through analysis of data on the characteristics and opinions of visiting nurses, patients, and human resources.[6]

An instrument and method for use in auditing records of public health nurses was developed by Phaneuf.[7] In this method records are reviewed after patient discharge, allowing for appraisal of care in relation to patient individuality.

More recently, the American Nurses' Association published standards for community nursing practice,[8] and the National League for Nursing developed a problem-oriented record keeping system for use in community health nursing agencies.[9] A systems control model has been developed for the planning and evaluation of community nursing services.[10] A model for quality assurance in nursing which has also been developed has potential for use in public health nursing.[11] A quality assurance project has been conducted by the Pennsylvania Assembly of Home Health Agencies in which a modified version of the Joint Commission on Accreditation of Hospitals' model was used.[12]

The public health nursing literature to date has some methods to determine need for service and benefits obtained and some models for quality assurance. Little was known about the "state of the art" of quality assurance as currently applied in public health nursing agencies.

A survey of a sample group of service agencies was conducted to document quality assurance activities and perceived needs. The procedure and findings of this survey are reported. Implications are discussed with the authors' recommendations for quality assurance in public health nursing.

STATEMENT OF PROBLEM

The problem addressed by this project was the lack of knowledge about the current activities and needs of public health nursing in quality assurance. A systematic identification and review of quality assurance efforts was needed to provide essential information for individuals and organizations concerned with quality assurance in public health nursing.

The purpose of this project is inherent in the project's research question: What is the status of and perceived needs for quality assurance in public health nursing? Subsequently, the Quality in Nursing Care Committee of the Public Health Nursing Section, American Public Health Association, raised the following questions:

1. What methods of evaluating quality of care are used in public health nursing?
2. What methods of quality care evaluation are seen as needed by public health nurses?
3. What aspects of quality care are seen by public health nurses as most important to be studied?
4. Is there a relationship between size of agency and methods used and/or described as needed?
5. What methods are under consideration by agencies for use in the future?
6. What are the employment and educational characteristics for the individual(s) responsible for setting standards and evaluating public health nursing?

7. Are there particular factors that are seen by public health nurses as influencing or potentially influencing the quality and evaluation of care?

Because of the nature of the questions raised, the Committee planned a descriptive study using a survey approach. Opinions as well as factual information were sought.

PROCEDURE

Selection of Study Group

The sample frame for this study was made up of service agencies which employed nurses for public health work. Included in this sample frame were local official, voluntary and combination nursing agencies, community health centers, home care agencies, local community-based categorical health programs, and state health agencies. Excluded from the study were school and occupational health programs not under the authority of local community or state health agencies.

The service agencies were purposefully selected by members of the Quality in Nursing Care Committee of the Public Health Nursing Section, APHA. The criteria used for the selection of agencies were geographic distribution, size of agency and type of service provided. No attempt was made to stratify the sample selection by agency type, size and geographic location. The committee members' knowledge about agencies which was currently known, or likely to have been developed, or worked with methods for the systematic evaluation of nursing practice and patient care was also a criterion for selection.

Questionnaire Development

The questionnaire (see Fig. 1) was developed by a subcommittee of the Quality in Nursing Care Committee. The purpose of the questionnaire was to gather broad knowledge about the status of quality assurance programs in relation to community health nursing practice. The questionnaire was made up of three parts: Part A was designed to gather information on type, size and geographic location of participating agencies and characteristics of persons completing the questionnaire; Part B sought information about the type of quality assurance practices currently in use, persons within agencies responsible for quality assessment associated with setting standards and reviewing practice, and recommendations for the future conduct of quality assurance programs; Part C was designed to elicit specific information about the methods currently used by agencies queried. The form of the questionnaire permitted participants to respond to open-ended, as well as forced-answer items.

FIGURE 1
Status of Quality Assurance Questionnaire

AMERICAN PUBLIC HEALTH ASSOCIATION
PUBLIC HEALTH NURSING SECTION

QUALITY IN NURSING CARE COMMITTEE QUESTIONNAIRE

Please check or describe as indicated in Parts A, B and C those items that are applicable to your setting. Additional comments can be written on the back of the last sheet. Your name and the name of the agency/institution in which you are employed are not requested. Individual responses will be kept confidential: only grouped data will be reported.

Please return the questionnaire in the enclosed envelope by _____ .
Thank you in advance for your help.

Part A—Identifying Information: Please check the responses that most closely describe you or your setting.

1. *Setting*
   _____ Home health agency
   _____ City or county health dept.
   _____ State health department
   _____ School of nursing
   _____ Outpatient department
   _____ State/national professional
              organization
   _____ Community health center
   _____ Other (specify)_____
   _____

2. *Population Primarily Served*
   _____ Urban
   _____ Rural
   _____ Suburban
   _____ Mixed
   _____ Other (specify)_____
   _____

3. *Geographic Location*
   _____ North
   _____ South
   _____ East
   _____ West
   _____ Midwest

4. *Size of Nursing Staff/Enrollment*
   _____ less than 5
   _____ 6 to 10
   _____ 11 to 20
   _____ 21 to 50
   _____ 51—100
   _____ 101—300
   _____ 301—500
   _____ over 500

5. *Type of Institution*
   _____ Official
   _____ Voluntary
   _____ Private
   _____ Other (specify)_____
   _____

6. *Your Primary Responsibilities*
   _____ Administration
   _____ Education
   _____ Clinical practice
   _____ Supervision
   _____ Research
   _____ Other (specify)_____
   _____

7. *Your Professional Identification*
   _____ Nursing
   _____ Medicine
   _____ Public health
   _____ Other (specify)_____
   _____

FIG. 1 (continued)

Part B – General Information on Methods Used and Needed: Please check or specify as indicated. More than one response may be checked.

1. Have you ever used any of the following *methods of evaluating the quality of care* given by community/public health nurses? No _____ Yes _____ (Please check below.)

  _____ a. Peer review
  _____ b. Supervisory review
  _____ c. Intra-agency review by medical or nursing advisory committee
  _____ d. Consumer review committee
  _____ e. Intradisciplinary review committee
  _____ f. Regional manpower planning committee
  _____ g. Outside consultant review
  _____ h. Record audits
  _____ i. Scales or indices of nursing care (agency developed or published)
  _____ j. Indices of health status of community or groups
  _____ k. Objective measurements of patient outcomes
  _____ l. Other (specify) _____

  If you have not checked any of the above, please complete the remainder of Part B. If you have checked any of the above, please complete Part B and also Part C.

2. Are you planning to develop any particular method(s) in the near future?
  No _____ Yes _____ (What kind?) _____

3. In what area(s) of community/public health nursing practice do you believe measurement(s) of quality of care should be developed?

  _____ a. Child health services
  _____ b. Maternal health services
  _____ c. School health services
  _____ d. Mental health services
  _____ e. Care to the ill
  _____ f. Occupational health services
  _____ g. Communicable disease
  _____ h. Services provided in specialized community facilities (i.e., housing for elderly, retarded, disabled, etc.)
  _____ i. Environmental health services
  _____ j. General home health services
  _____ k. Other (specify) _____

  Please briefly explain your reason(s) for area(s) checked _____

4. If instruments to measure the areas you checked were available, what aspect(s) of quality do you think should be measured?

  _____ a. Characteristics of *interaction* (verbal or nonverbal) between the nurse and patient.
  _____ b. *Structure* (i.e., number of clients per patient; available equipment, resources, inservice, etc.).
  _____ c. *Process* (i.e., the events that occur during the time span the nurse is in contact with patient).
  _____ d. *Decision making* abilities of the nurse.
  _____ e. *Outcome* (i.e., patient response over time to care provided).
  _____ f. Other (specify) _____

  Please give examples of aspect(s) checked. _____

FIG. 1 (continued)

5. If the tools you specified were available, would you:

_____ a. Be willing to pilot test or support pilot testing of them in your agency/institution.

_____ b. Incorporate or support incorporating them after pilot testing demonstrated their usefulness.

_____ c. Develop methods based on requirements for evaluation from National Health Insurance and/or PSRO Boards.

_____ d. Work toward developing other measures not yet available.

_____ e. Not use any additional tools.

_____ f. Other (specify) _____

_____

6. By title and educational preparation, who in your agency/institution is responsible for setting standards of nursing practice? _____

By title and educational preparation, who in your agency/institution is responsible for reviewing practice in accord with set standards? _____

Is this the same person?   No _____   Yes _____

What approximate percent of his/her time is spent reviewing nursing practice? _____

7. In your county/city, are there recent situations developing in any of the areas listed below that you believe may have an effect on the quality of community health nursing practice?

_____ a. Legal   _____ e. Nursing professional groups

_____ b. Political   _____ f. Recruitment practices

_____ c. Financial   _____ g. Manpower planning

_____ d. Other professional groups _____ h. Other (specify) _____

                                         _____

If so, please explain briefly any of these: _____

_____

Part C — Information on Methods of Quality of Care (see Part B, Item 1). For each method used, please respond to the following questions.

A. *Name of Method* and name and address of source where copy can be obtained. Are there reports of implementation of this method available? If so, where? (Please send two copies, if available).

B. Is there evidence or *validity* and/or *reliability* for this method?

C. *Purpose of method* (include advantages, disadvantages, problems in application, length of time to complete, how often used).

D. How is the *sample* for evaluation selected in this method?

E. Were individual or grouped data *reported to staff?* Was this measure useful to staff? How?

F. Are you aware of any potential legal issues that may *deter* efforts to use these quality of care methods? (For example, record confidentiality, potential for suit if method documents unsatisfactory care, conflicts with other health personnel who may be indirectly evaluated). Please identify issues and explain briefly.

G. Have consumers been involved in developing and/or evaluating services by these methods? If so, how?

Comments — Please make any additional comments you believe will be helpful to the Quality of Nursing Care Comittee. Add additional sheets if needed.

Data Collection

The identification of agencies for inclusion in the study, the distribution of questionnaires, and the coding of returned questionnaires were accomplished through the work of regional coordinators in four geographic areas of the country and their committee members. Regional committees identified the study group in each region based on a common criterion for inclusion.

After establishing the coding procedures, all questionnaires were coded and this coded information was transferred to Optical Scanning Forms. Completed Optical Scanning Forms and questionnaires were forwarded to one regional coordinator. The data on Optical Scanning Forms were transferred to a computer tape for analysis. To reduce the amount of errors which were undetected by previous procedures, data checks for legal values were performed by the computer and appropriate corrections were made prior to the data analysis. The major thrust of the data analysis was carried out through the use of descriptive statistics.

FINDINGS

The study findings are presented in two parts. Part 1 presents a description of the status of quality assurance as reported by service agencies and presents additional comments made by respondents. Part 2 presents an analysis of quality assurance methods received in response to the request on the questionnaire.

Part 1 — Status of Quality Assurance

Respondents. Over three-quarters (430) of the persons completing the questionnaire for service agencies identified themselves as nurses, and 17.7 percent of the persons identified themselves as public health professionals. The remaining respondents (5.1 percent) included physicians, administrators and planners. Persons completing the questionnaire were chiefly responsible for administrative activities within the agency. For those persons (425) identifying only one area of responsibility within the agency, over 69 percent were responsible for administrative activities. Responsibility for supervision activities was identified by 17.2 percent (73 individuals), and clinical practice activities was identified by 13.7 percent (58 persons).

When persons identifying multiple areas of responsibility were combined with those identifying single areas of responsibility within the agency, 62 percent (355) of the persons completing the questionnaire identified administration as an area of their job function. For this same group of respondents within the agency, only 9.5 percent (54) of the respondents identified education as their job function and education was usually reported in combination with other job responsibilities. Few people identified research as a single responsibility or a job function combined with other responsibilities.

Five hundred sixty-six service agencies participated in the study. The participating agencies represented both local and state agencies or institutions. Local agencies included city-county health departments, home care agencies, combination nursing services and special categorical programs. For this study group the largest number of agencies responding to the questionnaire was categorized as official and non-official local agencies (55.8 percent).

Over 52 percent of the agencies reported serving a population which was made up of urban, rural, and suburban residents. About 25 percent of the agencies reported serving only rural residents, and 19.2 percent of the agencies reported serving urban or suburban residents. Over 62 percent of the agencies employed a staff of 20 or less. The proportion of agencies having a staff of 20 or less did not vary significantly by agency type. However, official and categorical agencies reported having a very small staff size (less than 5) more frequently than combination and non-official agencies.

Agencies participating in this study were compared by region with agencies in the United States employing nurses for public health work.[13] Of the agencies in the United States, 3.8 percent are state agencies, whereas 12.5 percent of the agencies included in this study are state agencies. Official agencies are the major employer of nurses for public health work in the United States, and represent about 77 percent of the employing agencies. In the current study official agencies represent about 32.5 percent of the participants.

In comparing the regional distribution of agencies in this study with agencies in the United States, it can be said that for all regions the study group has a lower representation of official agencies and a higher proportion of state, non-official and combination agencies. Except for the Mountain and Pacific regions, a greater proportion of non-official agencies are reported for the study group. Except for the New England and Middle Atlantic regions, categorical programs have a higher representation in the study group compared to the proportional distribution of agencies in the United States.

Quality Assurance Methods. Respondents were asked to identify the quality assurance methods currently in use by the agency from a listing of 11 methods. The methods from which the respondents selected included practice review by various individuals or groups, record audit, measures of patient outcomes and health indices of groups. Among the agencies responding, 13.8 percent (78) reported no assessment method in current use. An additional 13.9 percent (79) of the agencies reported the use of only one method. The percentage of agencies reporting no quality assurance method in use was highest for categorical programs and lowest for combination agencies, 27.8 percent and 3.9 percent respectively. The proportion of official and non-official agencies reporting the use of four or five methods and staff size of less than 100, increased as the staff size of the agencies increased. This same trend was present for state agencies using three methods.

Supervisory and record audit were the two most commonly reported methods used for assessing quality of care. This was true regardless of the number of methods employed. Regional manpower committees and measures of the health status of groups were the least frequently reported assessment methods. When only one quality assessment method was reported in use, supervisory review was the most frequently reported. Only four of the agencies reporting one method in use indicated the measurement of patient outcomes or health status of groups as a means for assessing quality care. Almost 50 percent of the agencies reported two, three, or four methods in use. For these agencies, peer and supervisory review and record audit were the most frequently reported combinations of methods employed.

In considering the number of methods and type of quality assurance methods used, it is interesting to note that peer and supervisory review and record audit are the most common methods employed. Intra-agency, interdisciplinary, and consumer reviews were most often employed in combination with three or four methods. Regional manpower committees were the least used group for assessing quality care. Indices of nursing care, health status of groups, and measures of patient outcomes were seldom reported as methods used for determining quality. Only 30 percent of the agencies reported the use of these assessment methods. When these measures were reported in use by agencies, the measures were most frequently employed in combination with four or more methods (see Table 1).

The respondents were asked to comment on the type of evaluation tool utilized in the agency by naming the tool. Almost one-quarter of the respondents stated that they were using record audits, and of this number 8 percent (55) of the agencies specifically mentioned Phaneuf's audit.[14] Other types of tools identified by respondents were National League for Nursing Guidelines for Utilization, Home Health Care Agency Case Record Review, and scales or indices of nursing care.

Standards and Practice Review. Setting standards for practice is a prerequisite for a quality assurance program. In order to ascertain information about standard setting, respondents were asked to identify persons or committees responsible for setting practice standards for the agency. About 10 percent of the agencies reported no person(s) or committee reponsible for setting standards. Non-official agencies reported the smallest percentage of agencies; categorical programs reported the highest percentage of agencies without a designated person or committee responsible for the task.

All agency types were less likely to designate a person or committee responsible for standard setting if staff size was five or less members. For all agency types, except combination agencies, smaller agencies were most likely to invest the responsibility for standard setting with one individual, whereas larger agencies (staff size greater than 20) were more likely to assign the responsibility to more than one individual or special committees. Non-official and combination agencies, more frequently than all other agency types, place the responsibility for standard setting in more than one individual or committee.

TABLE 1
Number and Type of Quality Assessment Methods Currently in Use by Service Agencies Employing Public Health Nurses

		Number of Agencies	Peer Review	Supervisory Review	Intra-Agency Review	Consumer Review	Intra-Disciplinary Review	Record Audit	Indices of Nursing Care	Measures of Patient Outcomes	Health Status of Groups	Outside Consultant	Regional Manpower Committee	Other
One	N	79	4	31	6	3	—	24	—	3	1	3	—	4
	%	14.0	5.1	39.1	7.6	3.8	—	30.4	—	3.8	1.3	3.8	—	5.1
Two	N	91	24	56	10	1	8	48	2	6	2	14	2	9
	%	16	26.4	61.5	11.0	1.1	8.8	52.7	2.2	6.6	2.2	15.4	2.2	9.9
Three	N	100	40	69	31	12	24	73	11	9	5	21	—	5
	%	17.7	40.0	69.0	31.0	12.0	24.0	73.0	11.0	9.0	5.0	21.0	—	5.0
Four	N	95	58	91	45	10	31	67	17	16	6	27	—	12
	%	16.7	61.0	95.8	47.4	10.5	32.6	70.5	17.9	16.8	6.3	28.4	—	12.6
Five	N	55	37	48	34	6	32	45	10	15	6	26	5	11
	%	9.7	67.3	87.3	32.7	10.9	58.2	81.8	18.2	27.3	10.9	41.8	9.1	20.0
Six or more	N	68	57	64	37	30	43	65	19	34	8	37	5	17
	%	12.0	83.8	94.1	54.4	44.1	63.2	95.6	27.9	50.0	11.8	45.6	7.4	25.0
Zero	N	78	—	—	—	—	—	—	—	—	—	—	—	—
	%	13.8												
Total	N	566	220	359	163	62	138	322	59	83	28	128	12	58
	%	100.0	38.9	63.4	28.8	21.9	48.8	56.9	10.4	14.7	4.9	22.6	2.1	10.2

When one individual was identified with the responsibility for standard setting this person was usually the administrator. Only 14 agencies designated a practitioner or staff person responsible for this task. Sixteen agencies designated an advisory or nursing committee as the only group responsible for standard setting.

Administrative personnel, practitioners, and staff nurses were designated the responsibility for standard setting most frequently for those agencies reporting more than one person or committee responsible for the task. For official agencies, administrative staff and professional committees were the most frequently cited combinations.

The pattern for designating persons or committees responsible for reviewing practice was similar to the pattern for standard setting, except that agencies participating in practice review were slightly less than the number of agencies participating in standard setting. Also, more agency types involved practitioners or staff and committees in the review process than for standard setting (see Table 2).

In examining the educational preparation of individuals responsible for setting standards for practice, it was found that the largest proportion of persons were nurses with educational preparation at the master's level. There was some variation among agency types that involved these nurses in standard setting. Combination agencies reported the highest percentage of nurses with master's degrees, whereas state agencies reported the lowest proportion of nurses with master's preparation involved in standard setting.

The proportion of nurses with baccalaureate preparation was highest for official and non-official agencies. For 41 of the agencies these nurses were the only persons responsible for standard setting. These agencies represented 23.8 percent of all non-official and official agencies reporting.

Nurses with no formal education beyond an associate degree or diploma program made up the smallest proportion of the nurse group involved in standard setting. Although this percentage is seemingly low, nurses with no formal preparation in community health nursing were the only persons assigned the responsibility for standard setting by 24 agencies. One-half of these agencies were official agencies.

A comparison of the educational preparation of nurses reviewing practice and that of nurses responsible for setting standards showed that a lower proportion of nurses with master's degrees were involved in reviewing practice. This was true for all agency types except state agencies. A higher proportion of nurses with baccalaureate degrees and nurses with no formal preparation in community health were involved in reviewing practice. For 14 percent (22) of the agencies reporting, the only person responsible for reviewing practice had no formal education beyond the associate degree or diploma program. Another 19 agencies reported the one person responsible for reviewing practice was someone other than a nurse. The differences in the distribution of the educational preparation of nurses responsible for standard setting compared to those responsible for reviewing practice, may be attributed to the greater involvement of staff nurses and practitioners involved in reviewing practice.

TABLE 2
Responsibility for Review of Nursing Practice by Agency Type and Staff Size

		Responsible for Practice							
		Single Individual		Committee		None Identified		Total Agencies	
Agency Type	Staff Size	N	%	N	%	N	%	N	%
Local Official	5 or less	31	60.8	10	19.6	10	19.6	51	27.9
	6–20	26	36.6	36	50.7	9	12.7	71	38.8
	21–100	12	27.3	29	65.9	3	6.8	44	24.0
	100 +	1	5.9	13	76.5	3	17.6	17	9.3
Non-Official	5 or less	8	32.0	13	52.0	4	16.0	25	19.4
	6–20	20	33.3	37	61.7	3	5.0	60	46.5
	21–100	9	24.3	26	70.3	2	5.4	37	28.7
	100 +	3	42.9	4	57.1	—	—	7	5.4
Combination	5 or less	2	25.0	5	62.5	1	12.5	8	10.5
	6–20	12	32.4	18	48.7	7	18.9	37	48.7
	21–100	7	33.3	13	61.9	1	4.8	21	27.6
	100 +	1	10.0	9	90.0	—	—	10	13.2
Categorical	5 or less	11	32.3	8	23.5	15	44.2	34	37.8
	6–20	7	29.2	12	50.0	5	20.8	24	26.7
	21–100	4	26.7	9	60.0	2	13.3	15	16.7
	100 +	3	17.6	12	70.6	2	11.8	17	18.8
State	5 or less	4	23.5	5	29.4	8	47.1	17	26.1
	6–20	10	35.7	11	39.3	7	25.0	28	43.1
	21–100	—	—	12	92.3	1	7.7	13	20.0
	100 +	—	—	6	85.7	1	14.3	7	10.8
Agency/staff size unknown		—	—	—	—	—	—	23	4.1
Total		171	30.2	288	50.9	84	14.8	566	100.0

Influences on Quality Assurance. In order to determine factors influencing quality assurance programs, respondents were asked to identify those areas associated with recent events which occurred in their city or county and had an influence on quality assessment. The areas to which these recent events were to be assigned included financial, legal, political, professional groups, recruitment practices, and manpower planning.

Events associated with the financial area were reported most frequently. The political area was the second, and the legal area was the third most frequently reported area influencing quality assurance programs. Non-official agencies reported events associated with the areas of nursing and other professional groups more frequently than those areas associated with the legal area (see Table 3).

Although the questionnaire was not designed to elicit positive or negative effects of the events, 29 agencies did comment. The most frequently occurring

TABLE 3
Recent Events Occurring which Influence Quality Assurance Programs, Classified by Area and Agency Type

Agency Type	Total Areas Reported		Areas															Agency No. Response Rate[a]	
			Legal		Political		Financial		Professional Nursing Group		Other Professional Group		Recruitment Practices		Manpower		Other			
	N	%	N	%	N	%	N	%	N	%	N	%	N	%	N	%	N	%	N	R
Local Official (N = 184)	370	32.7	68	18.4	59	15.9	110	29.8	36	9.7	30	8.1	31	8.4	27	7.3	9	2.4	35	19.0
Non-Official (N = 132)	246	21.8	29	11.8	38	15.4	61	24.8	41	16.7	39	15.9	17	6.9	15	6.1	6	2.4	32	24.2
Combination (N = 77)	148	13.1	17	11.5	33	22.3	41	27.7	10	6.8	16	10.8	12	8.1	9	6.1	10	6.8	16	20.8
Categorical (N = 97)	189	16.8	31	16.4	29	15.3	42	22.2	24	12.7	17	9.0	16	8.5	24	12.7	6	3.2	32	33.0
State (N = 71)	174	15.4	25	14.4	33	18.9	41	23.6	20	11.5	15	8.6	13	7.5	18	10.3	9	5.2	10	14.0
Unidentified agencies (N = 5)	—	—	—	—	—	—	—	—	—	—	—	—	—	—	—	—	—	—	5	100.0
Total	1,127	100.0	170	15.1	192	17.0	295	26.2	131	11.6	117	10.4	89	7.9	93	8.3	40	3.5	130	230.0

[a]Rate per 100 agencies.

negative influence was identified with the financial area. Comments included statements about financial status and its negative effect on personnel retention/ recruitment and program development and maintenance. Other comments addressed the difficulty in providing continuing education for staff, problems associated with political internal conflicts in the community, concern about physicians' assistants, and worries about malpractice suits.

Another open-ended question was designed to ascertain the respondents' awareness of legal issues which may deter efforts directed toward the use of quality care methods. Approximately 57 percent (322) of the agencies responded to this question and 37 percent of these respondents stated they knew of no legal issues which would adversely affect the use of quality assurance methods. The responses indicating a potential influence due to legal issues varied considerably among respondents. The concern most frequently mentioned by the respondents addressed the issue of record confidentiality. Respondents indicated a need to protect the patient, reviewers, and agency. A few respondents specifically mentioned the availability of school records to parents and children as a potential deterrent. Other respondents indicated general concerns about changes in Medicare rules and expanding nursing roles, labor relations, and lack of proper malpractice insurance. In a few instances respondents stated legal issues associated with mental health clinics, teenagers attending family planning clinics, and problems associated with discharging a patient from service as adversely affecting the quality assurance program.

Quality Assurance Needs. For purposes of determining the direction for future work associated with quality assurance, respondents were asked to identify aspects of quality assurance which required study and the types of programs to which quality assurance methods might be applied. Three aspects of a health program are commonly considered in determining program quality: structure, process, and outcome. Structure refers to those aspects of quality most commonly reviewed by accrediting bodies. In this context, organization, personnel, and management procedures are included as part of structure. Process refers to those activities carried out by the provider for or in behalf of clients and includes interaction between clients and provider, and decision making in relation to care. Outcome refers to that aspect of quality which reflects what happens to clients because of service received. Included in outcome are client or community benefits.

Only 9.9 percent (56) of the agencies responding did not identify any aspect of quality which required study. Over 55 percent (316) of the agencies selected all three aspects—structure, process, and outcome—as requiring further study. The need for further study relating to process was identified by over 80 percent (455) of the agencies. Except for those agencies identifying only one aspect of quality requiring further study, outcome was identified as the second most important aspect of quality in need of study. For those agencies identifying only one determinant for study, outcome was identified as the most important. No agency reporting only one area for study identified structure. Structure was identified only in combination with one or more of the aspects of quality (see Table 4).

TABLE 4
Number and Type of Determinants of Quality Assurance in Need of Study as Indicated by Service Agencies

Number of Determinants Identified	Number of Agencies		Determinants							
			Process		Structure		Outcome		Other	
	N	%	N	%	N	%	N	%	N	%
One	85	15.0	30	6.6	—	—	50	11.4	5	13.1
Two	109	19.3	109	24.0	32	9.3	75	17.1	2	5.3
Three	287	50.7	287	63.0	286	82.9	286	65.0	2	5.3
Four	29	5.1	29	6.4	29	8.4	29	6.6	29	76.3
Zero	56	9.9	—	—	—	—	—	—	—	—
Total	566	100.0	455	80.4	347	61.3	440	77.6	38	6.7

Since process was identified as an aspect of quality by most agencies responding, the data were examined to determine the components of process which seemed to be most important to agencies. Two components, interaction and decision making, were identified. These process components were identified respectively by 46 percent (260) and 50 percent (284) of the agencies.

For purposes of identifying programs to which quality assurance methods needed to be applied, respondents were asked to select from a list of programs commonly associated with community health. Forty-four agencies did not identify a program, and 108 agencies identified six or more programs. Over 50 percent of the agencies identified three or more programs requiring the application of quality assurance methods.

Maternal and child health programs, including school health services and general home care programs, were the programs most frequently identified as needing the development of quality assurance methods. Over 50 percent of the agencies identified these two programs. Environmental and occupational health programs were reported least frequently by agencies as requiring the application of quality assurance methods. These programs were most frequently identified by those agencies indicating a need for the application of quality assurance methods to four or more programs. The low reporting of environmental and occupational programs may be attributed to the fact that few occupational facilities were included among the responding agencies.

Over 32 percent (184) of the agencies identified "other" as a program requiring the development of quality assurance methods. It is possible that programs such as drug abuse, battered child services, and specialized chronic disease services may have been considered in the "other" category. No data were available to determine the respondents' intent for using the "other" category.

An open-ended question directed toward eliciting additional comments from respondents which would be helpful in furthering the development of quality assurance in public health nursing services was asked. Approximately 22 percent of the respondents provided comments to this question. These responses supported this survey and the need for an adequate, effective tool to measure quality care. Repeated concerns were classified into three areas: (1) behavioral objectives, (2) Medicare and other third party payments, and (3) time needs for using quality assurance tools and the added paper work required. The comments are summarized as follows:

- Agency goals and objectives need to be stated in measurable terms.
- Job descriptions should reflect the agency objectives and expected nurse behaviors in relation to the level of nursing to be implemented.
- The development of behavioral objectives specific to process and outcome is needed.

Comments indicated that a great deal of time and energy was spent in meeting the demands of Medicare and Medicaid. Medicare was viewed as "doctor oriented" rather than oriented to health care issues most routinely encountered by consumers of public health nursing services. Because payment mechanisms established for Titles XVIII and XIX focus on the technical aspects of nursing, there was a critical need to identify and establish professional aspects of nursing. Nursing needs to be considered for third party payments, especially with the growing number of nurses practicing in the expanded role and with the revision of nurse practice acts by states.

Respondents stated that a usable, comprehensive tool to evaluate the quality of nursing care was needed. It must be pertinent, simple, effective, not too time consuming, and involve a limited amount of paper work. Standards of care should be written for each service provided. A definite need was educating the nurses to the importance of measuring quality. Evaluation was often perceived as a threat to nurses and only when that idea is removed will measurement methods be effective. The more the method of evaluation is incorporated into daily staff activity, the more meaningful it is to staff, and the greater the accuracy and validity of data collected.

Willingness to Develop Quality Assurance Programs. Agencies expressed a high degree of willingness to participate in furthering the development and implementation of quality assurance programs. Only 5.6 percent (27) of the responding agencies indicated they would not be willing to use additional methods if developed. One hundred agencies (21 percent) indicated that their participation in furthering the development of quality assurance methods would be limited to using new methods and tools after their utility had been satisfactorily demonstrated. All other agencies indicated their willingness to participate in developing or pilot testing methods and tools. About 10 percent (56) of the agencies reporting agreed to participate in developing methods and tools, pilot testing, and using newly developed tools and methods.

Agencies reporting only one activity for participation indicated a willingness to pilot test instruments and methods most frequently. However, it should be pointed out that relatively fewer non-official agencies than any other agency type indicated pilot testing as the only activity in which they were willing to participate. Non-official agencies more frequently expressed a willingness to participate in the development of new methods based on legislative regulations. This was true regardless of the number of activities in which they agreed to participate.

Part 2—Analysis of Methods Received

A total of 129 methods of evaluating quality of care were returned, as requested on the questionnaire, by 81 agencies. Most respondents who returned methods indicated that evaluation of care was done on a regular basis. Some respondents indicated that evaluations, particularly peer review, were voluntary and done on a sporadic basis. The methods returned by agencies varied widely. Nationally available tools were returned by 33 percent of the agencies. Two-thirds of these tools were the Home Health Care Agency Record Review, while the remainder were Phaneuf's tool for record audit. Approximately 25 percent (21) of the agencies returned locally developed record audit forms. The majority of these audit forms were developed to examine different aspects of the nursing process which were expected to be part of the care provided to patients. A few of the audit forms considered outcome of care, although predetermined standards and criteria had been established in only one instance.

Some agencies submitted consumer evaluation and problem oriented record forms, structural criteria for agency evaluations, activity counts, descriptive studies and encounter and caseload analysis forms as their methods for assessing quality care.

Forms for evaluating nurse performance were returned by 17 percent (14) of the agencies. These were developed locally to examine qualities or activities of nurses which required data collection obtained through interview and record audit or observations by supervisors, administrators, or peers. Forty-one percent of these performance forms examined qualities, activities, or skills exclusive of the nursing process, such as personality characteristics and professional qualifications.

Respondents were asked to evaluate the value of the methods used. Their comments reflected a belief that review is important to the general improvement of patient services. Positive comments indicated that the review process made staff more aware of what to record in records, promoted useful exchange of interdisciplinary perspectives (i.e., among the nurse and speech and occupational therapists, social workers, and consumers), facilitated the development of creative ideas, helped describe caseloads and determined the needs of the population served, offered experiences for nurses in objective writing, and provided the nurse with fresh viewpoints.

Negative comments indicated that methods available were too subjective and that use of multiple methods did not reduce subjectivity, there was a lack of standards on which to base methods, difficulties were encountered when evaluation of nursing care was done by non-nurses, methods were cumbersome and time consuming, methods were not useful with families with multiple problems, there was an absence of methods that evaluate outcomes of care, and the use of methods required a high degree of coordination.

IMPLICATIONS AND RECOMMENDATIONS

This study draws singular attention to the need for the development of quality assurance models, methodologies, and instruments which can be systematically utilized in a variety of agency types employing public health nurses. Agencies recognize the limitations of current practices in quality assurance in relation to the functional purposes of their specific health service. In addition, it is the exception rather than the rule that existing methods and procedures provide adequate data for direction in the overall improvement of public health nursing services in the community. The need for the further development of quality assurance is documented by the agencies, and reinforced by their willingness to participate in the development of methods and tools.

As evaluative research transects practice, education, and administration, individuals from these specialties need to be involved in the development and application of methods. Agencies endeavoring to assess quality of care need to consider many items, including sampling techniques; relationships among independent, dependent, and extraneous variables; methods of data analysis and interpretation; and instrument reliability and validity.

This survey revealed few nurses, based on job title and educational preparation, with research expertise involved in quality assurance programs. Although nurses with graduate preparation in nursing or public health were the single largest group responsible for reviewing practice and setting standards, the extent to which their formal education prepared them to explore new horizons of practice through the application of research methodology is open to question. The potential for the development of quality assurance methods and procedures for community health becomes more critical when consideration is given to the fact that nurses with a baccalaureate degree, an associate degree, or hospital diploma outnumbered the nurses with graduate preparation responsible for both setting standards and reviewing practice. The research base of these basic educational programs is minimal at best. Thus, if community health nursing services are to provide the consumer with appropriate accountability for service received, it seems appropriate that four actions be undertaken by service and educational institutions.

1. Nurse researchers employed by educational institutions work collaboratively in quality assurance programs of agencies.

2. Service agencies employ nurses with research competence for the purpose of developing and administrating quality assurance programs.

3. Educational institutions incorporate into present curricula, content relevant to assessing quality care to enable beginning practitioners to actively participate in quality assurance programs of agencies.

4. Nursing research by graduate students focus on agency needs in evaluation.

Findings of this study point to the need for a greater sharing of methods utilized for assessing quality care among agencies. This was especially true for agencies with a small staff size (less than five). Although agencies with small staff represent about 23 percent of the agencies surveyed, these agencies represented about 46 percent of the agencies reporting the use of no quality assurance method. These same agencies were not likely to have assigned a person or committee the responsibility for setting standards or reviewing practice.

It is perhaps unrealistic to consider the implementation of the same quality assurance programs for small agencies as those for larger agencies. Thus, models for assessment will need to consider those methodologies and instruments which are feasible for implementing in agenices with limited resources. Quality assurance programs will be achieved best by coordinating resources available to these agencies collectively.

The need for sharing among agencies is demonstrated further by the finding that only a small number of agencies surveyed were able to state the name of the instrument currently in use for measuring quality assurance. This finding implies the remaining agencies have developed instruments locally or to meet their specific needs. Most probably such instruments have not been evaluated for reliability or validity. Wider application of the instruments developed by the agencies could lead to a higher degree of reliability and validity in the measurement of quality care.

Another significant finding was the widespread use of such methods as peer and supervisory review and record audit. Although these methods have been given the greatest attention in the nursing literature, there is little indication that findings from these methods have been documented in patient or community outcomes. Furthermore, unless these methods are considered in relation to consumer review and health outcomes of groups the impact on community health care is likely to be ignored.

The need to develop outcome measures for public health nursing practice is demonstrated by the respondents' identification of outcome determinants as an area of need in quality assurance, and the fact that few agencies reported using measures of patient outcomes or health indices of groups in assessing quality care. The development of outcome measures will require considerable research, since outcome measures currently in use are non-specific to public health nursing practice. The development of outcome measures for public health nursing practice may require the rejection of the current systems used or proposed for classifying patient health problems since these systems are directed toward cure rather than prevention or health maintenance.

The single most frequently reported program in need of quality assessment reported in this survey was general home care services. Although this finding may be a bias of the study due to the selection of the study group, this recommendation warrants special attention. Serious consideration should be given to the adoption of the Tracer Method for Assessing Health Care services.[15] The use of this method for assessing quality care will require the identification of health care problems highly prevalent among clients. One such health problem may be the functional capacity of clients.

Implicit in the analysis of methods received in this survey is bewilderment with the complexity of quality assurance programs. This bewilderment may be attributed to the generalized nature of public health nursing practice and the lack of an organizing framework for assessing quality care. It is recommended that an organizing framework be adopted which will facilitate agencies to undertake quality assessment programs within the capacities of their limited resources.

The organizing framework must distinguish between different units of service: individual, family, and community. Within these units of services are different diagnostic realms, such as physical, psychosocial, environmental, and cognitive. There are many specific elements in each realm which must be assessed to determine the nursing diagnosis. All components of the nursing process, namely, assessment, planning, implementing, and evaluating must be applied to each realm and unit of service.

While the individual public health nurse implements the total nursing process in her caseload, whether that be composed of individuals, families, subgroups of the population or communities, the agency must also establish priorities on the many types of evaluation needed. The specific type of evaluation must flow from the philosophies and objectives of the agency as well as from immediate concerns. If the agency is committed to serving the health care needs of the community at large, the evaluation of who is and is not served and the accessibility of the service becomes as critical as the evaluation of the quality, quantity, efficiency, effectiveness, and cost of services rendered. Although the literature contains numerous instruments, models, and methodologies for all types of evaluation, few were found to be utilized by the study respondents.

Assessing quality of care by focusing on any one of the three components— professional competency, clients, community or population groups—to the exclusion of others requires consideration of the inherent assumptions. For example, focusing on staff competency assumes that if the service provided is of good quality, then there is necessarily a benefit to both the client and the community. This particular focus requires need, satisfaction, and acceptance as well as benefit. Focusing on the client assumes that the client is representative of the community or population group and may ignore differences among groups and their needs. Assessing quality care based on the community assumes that community problems are a collection of client problems.

Preliminary to an evaluation of the impact of public health nursing services, baseline data must be accumulated that identifies the extent of needs upon which public health nurses can impact. Measurable objectives must be written in relation to these needs. The literature provides examples of how needs can be identified and programs and personnel planned to meet those needs.

The major concern of the Committee is the absence of funds on national, state, and local levels from federal and private resources for the conduct of the fundamental research which precedes method development, and for actual development and testing of quality assurance methods. Currently, individual agencies have been almost exclusively left on their own in the development of quality assurance methods. Cross communication among agencies is imperative to avoid unnecessary duplication and promote exchange of both successful and unsuccessful efforts. An ongoing exchange mechanism also requires financial support. Inadequate financial support is presently the greatest inhibitor to the attainment of sound quality assurance methods in community health nursing.

ABOUT THE AUTHORS

Charlotte Januska, MN, RN, was Committee Chairman of the Project Task Force; Jane Engle, MPH, RN (now Jane E. Allen), was Regional Coordinator of the Project Task Force, and Jean Wood, PhD, RN, was Consultant to the Project Task Force.

REFERENCES

1. R. Freeman and M. Lowe, "A Method for Appraising Family Public Health Nursing Needs," *American Journal of Public Health,* 52(1) (1963), 47-52.

2. J. E. Mickey, "Findings of Study of Extra-Hospital Nursing Needs," *American Journal of Public Health,* 53(7) (1963), 1047-1057.

3. D. E. Roberts and H. H. Hudson, *How to Study Patient Progress* (Bethesda, MD: Division of Nursing, Public Health Service, U.S. Department of Health, Education & Welfare, 1964).

4. M. Highriter, "Nurse Characteristics and Patient Progress," *Nursing Research,* 18(6) (November-December 1969), 484-501.

5. W. L. Johnson and C. A. Hardin, *Content and Dynamics of Home Visits of Public Health Nurses, Part I* (New York: American Nurses' Association, 1962); *Part II* (New York: American Nurses' Association, 1969).

6. J. Holliday, *Public Health Nursing for the Sick at Home: A Descriptive Study* (New York: Visiting Nurse Service of New York, 1967).

7. M. C. Phaneuf, *The Nursing Audit: Profile for Excellence* (New York: Appleton-Century-Crofts, 1972).

8. *Standards of Community Health Nursing Practice* (Kansas City, MO: American Nurses' Association, 1974).

9. *Problem-Oriented Record System for Community Health Nursing* (New York: National League for Nursing, 1974).

10. M. C. Kauffman, M. H. Morris, and O. M. Henry, "Application of System Control Model for the Planning and Evaluation of Community Nursing Services," paper presented at the American Public Health Association Convention, New Orleans, November 17, 1975.

11. *Model for Quality Assurance* (Kansas City, MO: American Nurses' Association, 1975).

12. R. M. Berkoben, *Quality Assurance Project Report* (Pittsburgh, PA: Pennsylvania Assembly of Home Health Agencies, 1976).

13. Division of Nursing, *Surveys of Public Health Nursing, 1968-1972* (Bethesda, MD: Bureau of Health Manpower, Public Health Service, Health Resources Administration, U.S. Department of Health, Education & Welfare, 1973), p. 33.

14. Phaneuf, *The Nursing Audit.*

15. D. M. Kessner, *A Strategy for Evaluating Health Services Contrasts in Health Status, Vol. 2* (Washington, DC: Institute of Medicine, National Academy of Sciences, 1973).

Part 2

MATERNAL-CHILD HEALTH REPORTS

Effectiveness of Public Health Nurse Home Visits to Primarous Mothers and Their Infants

Violet H. Barkauskas

INTRODUCTION

Twenty years have passed since Roberts prodded public health nurses to explore the outcomes of their services to individuals and families.[1] A 1977 review of research in the field by Highriter indicated that many questions regarding service effectiveness have remained unanswered.[2] Because of current concerns about the cost-effectiveness of health services and appropriate utilization of professional nursing personnel, studies of service effectiveness are especially important and timely.

The home visit has been a major mechanism for the provision of public health nursing services to clients. The home has many advantages as a site for the receipt and delivery of health services. It is convenient for the client and family. For patients unable or reluctant to travel to other sites, the home may be the only

Reprinted with permission from *American Journal of Public Health,* 73 (May 1983), pp. 573-580, copyright © 1983, American Journal of Public Health.
This research was partially supported by a National Research Service Award, No. 5F31NU05H103, from the Department of Health and Human Resources, 1978-1980.

option for the receipt of any health services. The home is a setting controlled by the patient. It can be a comfortable, relaxed environment for the discussion of concerns and needs.

A major disadvantage of home services to health care providers, and ultimately clients, is the cost of such services. Costs include the home visitor's travel expenses, time wasted in uncompleted home visits when the client or family is not at home, and decreased efficiency because only one client or family can receive attention at a time.

Families in the childbearing and early childrearing phases of family development have been a major focus of public health nursing services. The health information and counseling needs of prenatal and postpartum women and their infants are well documented.[3] In response to these needs, public health nurses have provided services to young families in home and clinic settings since the turn of the century. These services still comprise a major portion of the overall nursing program in many official health agencies.

The few published studies of the effectiveness of public health nurse home visits to women during the childbearing and early postpartum periods for the purposes of general health promotion have yielded inconsistent, but generally negative, results.

Lowe utilized an experimental design with random assignment to determine if public health nurse home visits heightened the compliance and self-care practices of prenatal patients.[4] No differences in outcomes were observed between 28 home-visited and an equal number of not-home-visited subjects. The actual services provided to subjects were neither controlled nor documented.

A study by Yauger of the effects of community health nursing services on multiparous patients during the prenatal and postpartum periods indicated no difference between 21 visited and 26 control group families for health status, health behavior, and health knowledge variables measured 10 to 11 months postpartum.[5] Families in this study received the nursing services routinely provided by the study agency and a minimum of four home visits. As in the Lowe study, the actual services provided to subjects were neither controlled nor documented.

In contrast, Hall demonstrated that instruction focused on infant behavior during a home visit made several days after hospital discharge could have significant and beneficial effects on the primipara's perceptions of her newborn, measured at one month.[6] Hall's intervention was structured health teaching concentrated in areas related to the study's outcome variables. The total sample for this study was 30 mothers. Programs of focused and extended public health nurse home services to infants at risk for unexpected infant death and child abuse have also demonstrated effectiveness in reducing risk.[7]

The effectiveness of home visits, consisting of structured health teaching to expectant and postpartum families for various health promotion purposes by paraprofessional health care workers who provided services similar to those of public health nurses, has been studied by several investigators.[8] Findings from these studies, although inconsistent, have demonstrated a trend toward improved health outcomes when services were initiated prenatally and included frequent visits reestablished early in the postpartum period and extended throughout the first year.

The purposes of this study were: to document the nature of public health nursing services provided to postpartum families during home visits; and to determine if home visits to primiparous mothers and their infants in their homes by public health nurses facilitate the achievement of health outcomes at a higher level than would be expected without such visits.

MATERIALS AND METHODS

The study site was a county in a midwestern state in the United States, with a population of slightly more than one million residents. The participating public health nursing agency was a unit of the county's health department. In 1979, this nursing service had approximately 220 budgeted positions, including 80 public health nurses.

Criteria for the selection of mother-infant pairs into the study were:

- Delivery at the county hospital.
- First live birth for mother.
- Infant 2,000 grams or larger at birth.
- Infant living with mother.
- Neither infant or mother hospitalized since delivery for a condition noted at the time of delivery.
- No separation longer than 14 days of mother and infant since delivery.

Mothers selected for the study were characteristically in their late teens, unmarried, and not high school graduates. They initiated care early in the second trimester and had an average of 10 to 11 prenatal care visits. Infants had a mean birthweight of 3282 grams, and a mean five minute Apgar score of 8.8. None had congenital anomalies noted at birth (see also Table 2).

Data Sources

Birth certificates provided the following data: sex, birthweight, mother's age, race, marital status, and education, education of father, month in which prenatal care was initiated, number of prenatal visits. Apgar scores at one minute and five minutes, and complications of pregnancy, labor, and delivery.

Other information was solicited during an interview with the mother when the infant was 24-28 weeks of age and included: infant's primary care giver, size of household, and assistance given to mother during the postpartum period.

At this time, data regarding specific, dependent variables were also obtained reflecting health of mother, health of infant, utilization of services for health promotion, and mother's parenting practices.

The independent variable was routine public health nursing service provided in the homes of the subjects and over the telephone between home visits. The investigator did not manipulate the routine services in any way. Public health nursing records were reviewed to obtain information on services delivered.

Instruments

A Postpartum Interview Questionnaire (PIQ) was constructed to measure variables relating to the health and the health services utilization of the mother and infant, and the mother's parenting practices. Before use, this was pre-tested with five mothers to assess clarity of wording and acceptability of content, and minor revisions made.

In addition, the Home Observation for Measurement of the Environment (HOME) tool[9] was used to measure both the quality and quantity of social, emotional, and cognitive support within the home. This 45 binary choice item instrument involves both observational and interview questions which measure six factors within an infant's environment: emotional and verbal responsivity of the mother; avoidance of restriction and punishment; organization of the physical and temporal environment; provision of appropriate play materials; maternal involvement with the child; and opportunities for variety in daily stimulation. Elardo and others reported a consistent interrater agreement of 90 percent and predictive validity for the tool.[10] HOME scores at six months of age were significantly correlated with Stanford-Binet test scores measured at 54 months of age.[11]

Procedures

Birth certificates for a four-month period (October 1978 through January 1979) were reviewed to obtain an initial list of subjects who apparently met the first three subject selection criteria. Then, mothers' names were searched in the public health nursing services index files to screen for additional infants and mothers who did not meet the remaining study subject selection criteria and to determine if the mothers and infants had been referred to and received public health nursing services.

Because the screened list of 429 mothers was almost equally divided between white and black mothers, the sample was planned so that approximately half of the subjects would be from each racial group. The mothers were distributed among four sublists according to home-visited status and race. Using a random numbers table, the investigator selected one-third of the sample, 143 mother-infant pairs, for participation in the study. This percentage would achieve a sample of 120 with an anticipated 16 percent attrition rate.

Early in the study the investigator found that sample attrition, mainly because of inability to locate mothers, was averaging around 50 percent. Therefore additional mothers were randomly selected. A total of 256 mother-infant pairs were ultimately selected for the sample, including 146 pairs from whom data were not collected for various reasons and 110 pairs who were study subjects. The reasons for non-participation of 146 sample pairs are displayed in Table 1. Failure to establish contact with mothers for various reasons accounted for 75.9 percent of nonpartici-pation, while lack of mother's cooperation after contact was established accounted for only 17.2 percent of nonparticipation. Attrition was unequally distributed, being 51.5 percent for black mothers, 60.0 percent for white mothers, 14.8 per-cent for home-visited mothers, and 74.3 percent for not-home-visited mothers.

TABLE 1
Reasons for Nonparticipation of 146 Mother-Infant Pairs Selected for the Sample

Reason	Number of Mother-Infant Pairs	Percentage of Nonparticipants
Family had no phone and was not at home at visit attempt	30	20.6
Family moved to unknown address	28	19.2
Family not home for appointment for data collection or refused to participate	25	17.1
Family had a phone, unable to contact before infant too old	24	16.4
Given address incorrect	18	12.3
Family moved out of area	11	7.5
Mother-infant pair did not meet study subject selection criteria when reviewed at 6 months	6	4.1
Extra pairs in groups already filled at end of study	4	2.7
Total	146	99.9

Table 2 contains a comparison of summary statistics for various variables among the three population subgroups—those not selected for the sample, those selected for the sample but from whom data were not obtained, and the study subjects. As previously noted, racial composition was manipulated by the in-vestigator to obtain equal representation of black and white mother-infant pairs in the sample. Although the mean age was lowest for the subjects, there is less than one year's difference between the means for the oldest and youngest groups. Thus, despite the large attrition, study subjects were similar to the population from which they were drawn and attrition did not seem to be selective according to any of the measured variables.

TABLE 2
Comparisons of Demographic Characteristics among Population Subgroups[a]

	Mother-Infant Pairs			
Variable	Not in Sample (*n* = 173)	In Sample, not Subjects (*n* = 146)	Sample Subjects (*n* = 110)	Significance[b] of Difference
Male infants	50.0%	54.8%	54.5%	NS[j]
Black mothers[c]	38.2%	50.7%	58.2%	.003
Mean birthweight (grams)	3150.	3193.	3282.	NS
Mean age of mother (years)	18.7	19.1	18.2	.050
Mean years mothers' education	10.7	10.8	10.7	NS
Mean years fathers' education	10.7	11.1	10.7	NS
Married mothers[d]	28.2%	34.2%	24.5%	NS
Mothers with parity of 0000[e]	84.4%	84.2%	82.6%	NS
Mean gestational age when prenatal care initiated (months)	3.6	3.5	3.5	NS
Mean number of prenatal care visits	10.62	10.94	10.43	NS
Mean Apgar one minute (points)	7.3	7.6	7.5	NS
Mean Apgar five minutes (points)	8.8	8.8	8.8	NS
Complications of pregnancy	0.0%	0.0%	0.0%	NS
Concurrent illnesses with pregnancy	0.0%	0.0%	0.9%[h]	NS
Complications of labor and delivery	0.6%[f]	4.8%[g]	3.7%[i]	NS
Congenital anomalies	0.0%	0.0%	0.0%	NS

[a] Population refers to births in the county hospital between October 1, 1978 through January 31, 1979 meeting study sample selection criteria.
[b] Determined by ANOVA or chi-square methods.
[c] Remainder white.
[d] Remainder unmarried.
[e] Indicates no previous pregnancies.
[f] One case, Cesarean section (CS).
[g] One case, fetal distress; 6 cases, CS; 1 case, breech presentation.
[h] One case, premature rupture of membranes.
[i] Four cases, CS.
[j] Not significant at the .05 level.

The distribution of study subjects by public health nurse visit and race variables is displayed in Table 3.

Multivariate contingency table and two-way analysis of variance techniques were the primary methods used to analyze data.

RESULTS

A number of variables were significantly related to race. Black mothers were significantly younger, better educated, more apt to be involved in work or school. They were more likely to reside in larger households and less likely to be married than white mothers. It is important to note that no significant public health nursing

TABLE 3
Distribution of Study Mother-Infant Pairs by Home-Visit Status and Race

| | Home-Visit Status | | |
Race	Home-Visited	Not-Home-Visited	Total
Black	35	29	64
White	32	14	46
Total	67	43	110

visit effects, which might indicate selection criteria for home visits, were observed among the descriptive variables.

A total of 48 nurses provided the public health nursing services to study subjects. The nurses' mean age was 35.9 years, with a median age of 31 years. Typically nurses were white and female; they had a median of seven years' total nursing experience, and a median of two years' public health nursing experience. Seventy-seven percent had at least a baccalaureate degree.

Public health nurses had a total of 236 completed and attempted contacts with the 67 families in the home-visited group. Of these 236 contacts, 143 (60.6 percent) were completed home visits, 49 (20.8 percent) were telephone calls, and 44 (18.7 percent) were attempted home visits for which the mother was not home. The 35 black families who were visited received an average of 2.08 home visits per mother-infant pair; and the 32 white families visited received an average of 2.18 home visits per family. The average age of black infants at the first contact with a public health nurse was 3.17 weeks, and for white infants was 3.32 weeks. However, over half of initial contacts were made during the first two postpartum weeks.

Table 4 displays the services provided during 192 completed home visits and telephone calls. Assessment of mother, infant, and family services predominated in frequency when compared to frequencies of intervention and treatment services. Use of health services is the most frequently performed assessment activity in behalf of both mothers and infants. Instructions predominated as the primary interventions of the public health nurses with diet, child care, use of health services, and feeding methods the predominant instruction topics.

Of the 65 home-visited mothers who answered the question: "Were the public health nursing visits helpful to you?" 56 (86.2 percent) responded that the visits were helpful and 9 (13.8 percent) responded that the visits were not helpful. The subjects' perceptions of what was helpful in the public health nursing visits indicated that information-giving was the major type of assistance (Table 5).

Group data for many of the dependent variables are summarized in Table 6 with results of significance tests for effects of race and of public health nursing visit. Only one of the 18 variables demonstrated significant PHN effect: home-visited mothers were more apt to express concerns about health matters than not-home-visited mothers. Neither self-estimation of health nor use of birth control differed significantly by PHN visit or race. However, white mothers were more likely to report the presence of postpartum health problems, but less likely to have a postpartum examination than black mothers. Three of four white mothers who reported a second pregnancy had received PHN home visits.

TABLE 4
Services Provided to Study Subjects during Completed Home Visits and Telephone Contracts[a]

Service	Frequency	Percent of Completed Contacts in Which Service Occurred	Rank[b]
Assessment of mother			
Health services use	79	41.1	3.5
Physical status	76	39.6	5
Family planning practices	62	32.3	7
Plans for work/school	59	30.7	8
Mothering skills	53	27.6	9
Self-care practices	42	21.9	14.5
Health history	34	17.7	18
Support systems	33	17.2	19
Psychological status	27	14.1	22
Assessment of infant			
Health services use	107	55.7	1
Diet	99	51.6	2
Physical status	79	41.1	3.5
Development	65	33.9	6
Method of feeding	46	24.0	12
Health history	46	24.0	12
Sleep	30	15.6	20.5
Assessment of family			
Relationships	46	24.0	12
Finances	42	21.9	14.5
Environment	36	18.8	17
Dynamics	6	3.1	
Instructions			
Diet-general	47	24.5	10
General child care, including growth and development information	40	20.8	16
Use of health services	30	15.6	20.5
Feeding methods for infant	10	5.2	
Re-instruction of instructions of others	9	4.7	
Safety	8	4.2	
Social, cognitive, growth fostering activities for infant	8	4.2	
Use of thermometer	7	3.6	
Family planning	6	3.1	
Other areas of instruction (11 areas noted 1-5 times each)	27	14.1	
Follow-up of problems			
Positive gonorrhea culture	3	1.6	
Emergency room visit	3	1.6	
Referrals			
To well-child clinic	10	5.2	
Other referrals to six types of services noted 1-5 times each	18	9.4	
General supportive interactions	17	8.8	
Miscellaneous activities			
Inform about resources	9	4.7	
Other miscellaneous activities (six activities noted 1-5 times each)	19	9.9	

[a] $N = 192$

[b] Only individual items at a frequency of greater than 20 are ranked.

TABLE 5
Respondents' Replies to Question Regarding Ways in which Public Health Nursing Visits Were Helpful[a]

Response	Frequency[b]
Provided information, or taught generally or specifically about: feeding, diet, thermometer reading, eye care, babies' cries, handling babies, child care, clinic visits, resources	56
Checked baby, navel, circumcision	12
Provided availability to a health care provider	11
Provided general support, reassurance	6
Heightened awareness of health	3
Helped to obtain things	1

[a] $N = 56$
[b] Column total is greater than 56 because some respondents provided two responses.

No significant PHN visit effects were noted for home scores. Black mothers demonstrated lower total home scores than white mothers, $F(1,107) = 14,468$, $p < .01$.

DISCUSSION

Only one statistically significant difference in health outcome was observed between home-visited and not-home-visited mother-infant pairs: home-visited mothers were more likely to express health concerns than not-home-visited mothers. Since this was only one of more than 18 variables examined, chance itself could account for the statistical significance.

An incidental finding is the differential in health assets and deficits between the study's two racial groups despite their similar economic status and health system experience. Findings for white mothers reflect a theme of illness and lack of compliance. Black mothers reflect needs relating to several basic mothering skills.

The finding of no difference between home-visited and not-home-visited families for most dependent variables could be related to limitations in the study's methodology, the public health nursing services provided to study subjects, or the basic structure of public health nursing services for families.

A major limitation of the study's methodology was the lack of random assignment to treatment and comparison groups and the concomitant lack of control over services provided to mother-infant pairs. This limitation was necessitated by ethical concerns of agency personnel regarding the denial of services to families ordinarily receiving them, a concern not unique to public health nursing settings and identified as a major objection to experimentation in many types of human services.[12] Nevertheless, the random selection process seems to have selected a group of subjects similar to the population except for the investigator-manipulated,

TABLE 6
Dependent Variable Data Summary (n = 110)

| | Percentages | | | | Effects[a] | |
| | Home-Visited | | Not-Home Visited | | | |
Variable	Black (n = 35)	White (n = 32)	Black (n = 29)	White (n = 14)	PHN Visit	Race
Mother's health and health services utilization variables						
Mother's health					NS[b]	NS
Very good	45.7	25.0	34.5	35.7		
Good	40.0	46.9	51.7	57.1		
Fair	14.3	28.1	13.8	7.1		
Postpartum health problems					NS	**
Yes	22.9	59.4	24.1	35.7		
No	77.1	40.6	75.9	64.3		
Use of birth control					NS	NS
Yes	74.3	65.6	65.5	57.1		
No	25.7	34.4	34.5	42.9		
History of postpartum examination					NS	*
Yes	91.4	71.9	93.1	85.7		
No	8.6	28.1	6.9	14.3		
Satisfaction with mothering					NS	NS
Very/quite satisfied	97.1	71.9	86.2	100.0		
Moderately satisfied	2.9	21.9	6.9	0.0		
Not too satisfied/unsatisfied	0.0	6.2	6.9	0.0		
Satisfaction with baby					NS	NS
Very/quite satisfied	100.0	90.6	93.1	100.0		
Moderately satisfied	0.0	9.4	6.9	0.0		
Concerns about health					*	NS
Yes	41.2	50.0	20.7	28.6		
No	58.8	50.0	79.3	71.4		
Infant health and health services utilization variables						
Infant's health					NS	NS
Very good	54.3	59.4	31.0	57.1		
Good	40.0	34.4	58.6	35.7		
Fair	5.7	6.2	10.3	7.1		
Well-child clinic visits					NS	NS
0-3	42.4	44.8	26.9	54.5		
4 or more	57.6	55.2	73.1	45.4		

Received second DPT and polio immunization					
Yes	75.0	88.5	89.3	53.6	NS NS
No	25.0	11.5	10.7	36.4	
Illness visits to clinic					
0-1	68.6	40.6	58.6	28.5	NS **
2 or more	31.4	59.4	41.4	71.4	
Total number of health problems					
0-1	25.7	21.9	31.0	42.9	NS NS
2-3	54.3	53.1	44.8	50.0	
4 or more	20.0	25.0	24.1	7.1	
Parenting variables					
Infant's primary caregiver					
Mother	85.7	96.9	89.7	100.0	NS *
Other	14.3	3.1	10.3	0.0	
Uses appropriate type of milk[c]					
Yes	87.9	71.9	82.8	64.3	NS *
No	12.1	28.1	17.2	35.7	
Uses appropriate diet[d]					
Yes	52.9	53.1	51.7	50.0	NS NS
No	47.1	46.9	48.3	50.0	
Uses thermometer					
Yes	65.5	75.0	57.7	92.9	NS **
No	34.5	25.0	42.3	7.1	
History of accident					
Yes	48.6	65.6	65.5	42.9	NS NS
No	51.4	34.4	34.5	57.1	
Number of accidents					
None	51.4	34.4	34.5	57.1	NS NS
1	25.7	34.4	24.1	21.4	
2 or more	22.9	31.2	41.4	21.4	

* $p < .05$.
** $p < .01$.
[a] Determined by multivariate contingency table analyses.
[b] $p > .05$.
[c] Breast milk or iron fortified formula.
[d] Daily consumption of 0-2 servings of cereal, 0-1 slice of toast, 0-½ jar of meat, 1 jar of fruit or vegetable, and 24-32 oz. of appropriate milk; minimal use of table foods; and no routine use of snack foods.

race characteristic (Table 2). The sample selection and attrition processes did not appear to be biased by any variable documented on the birth certificates which were a useful source of information for descriptive and comparative data.

Nonparticipation was large, and the investigator probably collected data from the more stable and receptive of the mothers chosen for the sample. Thus the overall data may be biased in a positive direction. It is also possible that the home-visited families were at greater risk for health problems than the not-home-visited families. The finding of little difference at six months postpartum may indicate that home-visited families were brought to levels of health and functioning comparable to the hypothetically low-risk, not-home-visited families. Nevertheless, the lack of PHN visit effect for the descriptive variables noted on birth certificates and the lack of specification of reasons for home-visit service selection on the family records weaken this argument. Low-income, primiparous mothers were considered high-risk by the study agency, and evidence exists that home visits were unsuccessfully attempted with many of the families in the not-home-visited group.

Although the young, primiparous, low-income mother can be classified as being at increased risk,[13] study data suggest that not all such mothers need or benefit from public health nurse home visitation. Future studies to determine specific risk factors which would identify primiparous mothers who need and would benefit from home visits are indicated.

Over three-fourths of the nurses who provided the study interventions were prepared at the baccalaureate or higher level, reflecting a higher educational level than the national figure of approximately 41 percent in 1977.[14] It is therefore reasonable to assume that the potency of the interventions was as optimal as that in public health nursing practice nationally.

Descriptions of PHN services were obtained from recordings and are consequently subject to the limitations of records as accurate data sources. The recorded services provided to study subjects reflected a nursing process with a major emphasis on assessment. A home visit only for assessment does not meet cost-effectiveness criteria for screening techniques. Perhaps screening by nurses working with mothers and families in antenatal clinics, postpartum units, and postpartum clinics could be used more effectively and systematically in the identification and referral of high-risk mothers.

Instruction appears to be the primary intervention of public health nurses with well mothers and infants. One-on-one teaching is a very expensive instructional modality. Group instruction is an alternative and can be as effective as individual instruction.[15]

The expectant or postpartum mother and her infant are usually in a period of intense involvement with health care providers and systems. In most cases, the home visit is supplementary to primary care services provided in another setting and often by others. Although public health nurses have established comprehensive health goals for their services to families, these goals may need focus and specification for individual families.

Public health nursing interactions in the home are a very small part of the lives of the mother-infant pairs served. Considering the amounts of energy and time which change and learning require, the expectation of major achievements from interactions lasting up to several total hours may be unreasonable. The study outcome of heightened health concern may be a realistic goal for such short-term services to well families.

The need for further evaluative research of public health nursing services, especially those for preventive purposes, is a major recommendation for future research. Because of limitations on the findings of quasi-experimental designs, research should utilize as controlled a design as possible within the field setting in order to fully maximize the benefits of random assignment.

Descriptive research is indicated as well. Only a small amount of data have been published regarding the characteristics of the populations actually being served by public health nurses and the interventions being utilized by them.

Public health nurses can no longer afford to look upon the home visit as a general, therapeutic event. The specific goals and interventions of home visits must be determined if this practice is to be scientifically and financially justified.

ABOUT THE AUTHOR

Violet H. Barkauskas, PhD, RN, CNM, is Director of Research, National Center for Homecare Education and Research, and Associate Professor, Community Health Nursing, School of Nursing, University of Michigan, Ann Arbor. The author acknowledges the assistance of Drs. Shu-Pi Chen and Deborah Oakley in critiquing earlier drafts of this paper.

REFERENCES

1. D. E. Roberts, "How Effective is Public Health Nursing?" *American Journal of Public Health,* 52 (1962), 1077-1083.

2. M. E. Highriter, "The Status of Community Health Nursing Research," *Nursing Research,* 26 (1977), 183-192.

3. E. R. Benson and J. Q. McDevitt, *Community Health and Nursing Practice* (2nd ed.; Englewood Cliffs, NJ: Prentice-Hall, 1980); S. N. McCabe, "Anticipatory Guidance for Families with Infants," in D. H. Hymovich and M. U. Barnard, eds., *Family Health Care: Developmental and Situational Crises,* Vol. 2 (New York: McGraw-Hill, 1979); and U.S. Department of Health, Education, and Welfare, *Healthy People: The Surgeon General's Report on Health Promotion and Disease Prevention* (Washington, DC: Government Printing Office, 1979).

4. M. L. Lowe, "Effectiveness of Teaching as Measured by Compliance with Medical Recommendations," *Nursing Research,* 19 (1970), 59-63.

5. R. A. Yauger, "Does Family Centered Care Make a Difference?" *Nursing Outlook,* 20 (1972), 320-323.

6. L. A. Hall, "Effect of Teaching on Primiparas' Perception of Their Newborn," *Nursing Research,* 29 (1980), 317-321.

7. R. G. Carpenter and J. L. Emery, "Identification and Follow-Up of Infants at Risk of Sudden Infant Death in Infancy," *Nature,* 250 (1974), 729; and C. H. Kempe, "Child Abuse: The Pediatrician's Role in Child Advocacy and Preventive Pediatrics," *American Journal of Diseases of Children,* 132 (1978), 255-260.

8. E. Siegel, K. E. Bauman, E. S. Schaefer, et al., "Hospital and Home Support During Infancy: Impact on Maternal Attachment, Child Abuse and Neglect, and Health Care Utilization," *Pediatrics,* 66 (1980), 183-190; and C. P. Larson, "Efficacy of Prenatal and Postpartum Visits on Child Health and Development," *Pediatrics,* 66 (1980), 191-197.

9. R. H. Bradley and B. M. Caldwell, "Early Home Environment and Changes in Mental Test Performance in Children from 6 to 36 Months," *Developmental Psychology,* 12 (1976), 93-97; and R. Elardo, R. Bradley, and B. M. Caldwell, "The Relation of Infants' Home Environments to Mental Test Performance from Six to Thirty-Six Months: A Longitudinal Analysis," *Child Development,* 46 (1975), 71-76.

10. Elardo, Bradley, and Caldwell, "The Relation of Infants' Home Environments to Mental Test Performance."

11. Bradley and Caldwell, "Early Home Environment and Changes in Mental Test Performance in Children."

12. H. W. Reicken and R. F. Boruch, eds., *Social Experimentation: A New Method for Planning and Evaluating Social Intervention* (New York: Academic Press, 1974).

13. H. C. Chase, ed., "A Study of Risks, Medical Care and Infant Mortality," *American Journal of Public Health* (supplement), 63 (1973), 1-56.

14. *Facts about Nursing: 1980-81* (Kansas City, MO: American Nurses' Association, 1981).

15. H. J. McNeil and S. S. Holland, "A Comparative Study of Public Health Nurse Teaching in Groups and in Home Visits," *American Journal of Public Health,* 62 (1972), 1629-1637.

A Randomized Clinical Trial of Early Hospital Discharge and Home Follow-up of Very-Low-Birth-Weight Infants

Dorothy Brooten, Savitri Kumar, Linda P. Brown,
Priscilla Butts, Steven A. Finkler, Susan Bakewell-Sachs,
Ann Gibbons, and Maria Delivoria-Papadopoulos

More than 230,000 low-birth-weight infants are born annually in the United States, and more than 36,000 of these infants weigh less than 1500 g.[1] In addition, the proportion of live births made up by infants weighing less than 1500 g has changed little in the past several decades.[2] Although advances in neonatal intensive care have been credited with reducing mortality and morbidity in this group,[3] recent studies suggest that the environment of the neonatal intensive care unit—with its bright lights and high noise levels—may have a permanent adverse effect on an infant's hearing, vision, and motor coordination.[4] Prolonged hospitalization increases the infant's chances of contracting infections and has been associated with failure to thrive, child abuse, and parental feelings of

Reprinted with permission from *The New England Journal of Medicine,* 315 (October 9, 1986), pp. 934-939, copyright © 1986, The New England Journal of Medicine.
This study was supported by a grant (6742) from the Robert Wood Johnson Foundation and a grant (5-R21-NU0082) from the Division of Nursing, Health Resources Administration, U.S. Department of Health and Human Services.

inadequacy.[5] Hospital care for these infants is one of the most expensive of all types of hospitalization.[6] Despite initial hospital expenditures averaging up to $167,000 for very-low-birth-weight infants,[7] formalized home care services are almost completely lacking after these infants are discharged. This lack of services is particularly troubling since this group is at high risk for failure to thrive, problems associated with chronic lung disease, anemia, seizures, and developmental delays, as well as parenting problems.[8] In the first year of life, the rate of rehospitalization for very-low-birth-weight infants is four times the rate for normal-birth-weight infants (2500 g or more) and their postneonatal death rate is five times as high.[9] Compounding these problems, a disproportionate number of very-low-birth-weight infants are born to poor, young mothers with questionable resources to provide adequate care after discharge.[10]

Although home visits by nurses have been used in a variety of medical specialties to improve care and decrease health care costs, the efficacy of visits by perinatal nurse specialists to very-low-birth-weight infants after discharge has not been documented. This clinical trial was undertaken to examine whether it is safe and economical to discharge very-low-birth-weight infants (1500 g or less) early if they meet certain conditions and to subsidize home care services with any savings that result from shorter hospitalizations.

METHODS

Infants with birth weights of 1500 g or less who were born at the Hospital of the University of Pennsylvania between October 1982 and December 1984 were randomly assigned to one of two groups, after their parents gave informed consent to their participation in the study. Infants in the control group were discharged according to routine nursery policy, which required that the infant be clinically well, feeding well, and weigh approximately 2200 g. Although parents received support and instruction from nursery nurses about their infant and his or her care after discharge, no routine home follow-up care by nurses was provided for this group.

Infants in the early-discharge group were discharged before they weighed 2200 g so long as they met the following criteria: (1) they were clinically well and able to feed by nipple every four hours; (2) they were able to maintain their body temperature in an open crib in room air; (3) no evidence of serious apnea or bradycardia was found in a 12-hour recording of the infant's heart rate and respiration; (4) the mother or other caretaker demonstrated satisfactory care-taking skills; and (5) the physical home environment and facilities for the care of the infant were adequate.

Infants and families in the early-discharge group received home follow-up care provided by a nurse. Since specialty practice in the care of these high-risk infants and their families formally occurs at the master's degree level in nursing, one full-time nurse and two part-time relief nurses with master's degrees in perinatal and neonatal nursing were hired to provide follow-up care to the families. A nurse specialist contacted one or both parents soon after the infant's birth and at least once a week during the infant's hospitalization to promote the parents' interaction with the infant; to evaluate the parents' perceptions and concerns about the infant; to teach parents to bathe, handle, and soothe the infant, to take his or her temperature, and to prevent infection; and to provide information about the infant's sleeping patterns, differences in infant temperature, reportable signs and symptoms, and times for routine medical care. Weekly contact with parents helped to establish a rapport between parents and the nurse specialist and provided continuity for the parents as the infant was transferred from the intensive care unit to the intermediate care unit and then home.

Before discharge, parents were required to demonstrate satisfactorily the basic care-taking skills described above and a basic knowledge of any medications or special procedures required in the infant's care. Approximately one week before discharge, the nurse specialist made a home visit to coordinate planning for the discharge and to evaluate the adequacy of heat in the home, the safety of the environment, and the adequacy of facilities for the care of the newborn. When problems were encountered, the nurse specialist consulted with physicians, hospital social-service personnel, and others in the community.

After the infant was discharged, the nurse made home visits during the first week and at 1, 9, 12, and 18 months. The visits included a physical examination of the infant, developmental screening, confirmation of appointments for medical follow-up care, an assessment of the parents' coping ability and care-taking skills and support systems, and instruction and counseling regarding infant care and infant stimulation, if needed. The nurse was in contact with the parents by telephone at least three times a week for the first two weeks after discharge and weekly thereafter for eight weeks. The nurse specialist was on call from 8:00 a.m. to 10:00 p.m. Monday through Friday and from 8:00 a.m. to noon on weekends, to respond to parents' concerns and special problems. Medical backup for the nurse was provided by neonatologists at the hospital. Long-term medical follow-up care for infants in both groups was provided either by the hospital's high-risk follow-up clinic or by private pediatricians.

Infants with life-threatening congenital anomalies, grade 4 intraventricular hemorrhage, extensive surgical intervention, oxygen dependence for a period of more than 10 weeks, or a combination of these factors were excluded from the study.

Sample

Of 136 infants eligible for enrollment at birth, 57 were not included in the study because of death (6 infants), the complications described above as reasons for exclusion (34), family complications (7), or their parents' refusal to participate (10). The sample included 72 mothers and 79 infants: 36 mothers and 39 infants (3 sets of twins) in the early-discharge group, and 36 mothers and 40 infants (4 sets of twins) in the control group (Table 1). There were no statistically significant differences between the groups in terms of the mother's age, educational level, marital status, race, or number of children; the family structure; the availability of a telephone in the home; the type of transportation available in an emergency; the family's reported annual income; the type of

TABLE 1
Characteristics of Very-Low-Birth-Weight Infants and Their Families

Characteristic	Early-Discharge Group	Control Group
Mother		
Number	36	36
Mean age ± SD (range)	24 ± 7 yr (16-44)	23 ± 6 yr (12-38)
Education level		
Less than high school	42%	30.5%
High school	28%	39.0%
More than high school	30%	30.5%
Marital status		
Married	31%	33%
Unmarried	69%	67%
Race		
Black	83%	78%
White	17%	22%
Family		
Hospital insurance		
Medicaid	75%	56%
Private	25%	44%
Income		
$5,000 or less	34%	26%
$5,001–9,999	43%	32%
$10,000–49,000	17%	26%
$50,000 or more	6%	16%
Infants		
Number	39	40
Mean birth weight ± SD (range)	1187 ± 198 g (740–1490)	1148 ± 203 g (710–1500)
Mean gestational age at birth ± SD (range)	30 ± 2 wk (26–37)	30 ± 2 wk (26–37)

health insurance; or the number of children under 5 years of age (a variable associated with increased infection rates among low-birth-weight infants after discharge). Although no data on living conditions were gathered on the control group, inadequate heating, food, and formula were problems during follow-up for 11 percent of the families in the early-discharge group.

There were no statistically significant differences between the groups in terms of the infants' mean birth weight, gestational age, appropriateness of size for gestational age, number of days of ventilation, or number of days spent in the intensive care nursery. Seventy infants were of appropriate size for gestational age at birth, whereas nine infants were small for gestational age (four in the early-discharge group and five in the control group). Ninety-seven percent of the infants had complicating conditions while they were hospitalized; these included respiratory distress syndrome (30 in the early-discharge group and 35 in the control group); necrotizing enterocolitis (2 in each group); surgery (1 in each group); and jaundice requiring phototherapy (37 in the early-discharge group and 39 in the control group).

Twenty-five infants (32 percent) were discharged with apnea monitors (14 in the early-discharge group and 11 in the control group). Fifty-nine infants (75 percent) were discharged with medications such as theophylline or vitamin E to be administered at home by their parents (28 in the early-discharge group and 31 in the control group). Because of the time limits of the study, 12 infants, 6 in each group, were followed for less than 18 months.

Statistical Analysis

All data are expressed as means $\pm$ SD. The significance of differences was determined by unpaired t-tests.

RESULTS

Infants in the early-discharge group were discharged from the hospital a mean of 11.2 days earlier, weighed 200 g less, and were approximately two weeks younger at discharge than the infants in the control group (Table 2). The difference in the average length of hospital stay between the groups was statistically significant ($p < 0.05$).

There were no statistically significant differences between the groups in terms of the number of rehospitalizations, the number of acute care visits, the incidence of failure to thrive, reported child abuse, or foster placement during the 18-month follow-up period. The two cases of reported child abuse in the early-discharge group were in families that did not comply with requirements for medical follow-up during the child's second year of life. Infants in two of the four families in the control group in which child abuse was reported were

TABLE 2
Characteristics of Very-Low-Birth-Weight Infants at Discharge and during Follow-up

Characteristic	Early-Discharge Group (N = 39)	Control Group (N = 40)
Mean days of hospitalization ± SD (range)	46.5 ± 12.5[a] (20–79)	57.7 ± 17[a] (21–94)
Mean weight at discharge ± SD (range)	2072 ± 131 g (1880–2500)	2280 ± 179 g (1980–2650)
Mean gestational age at discharge ± SD (range)	36 ± 2 wk (34–39)	38 ± 2 wk (34–44)
Number of infants rehospitalized		
Within 14 days	4	5
Within 18 months	10	10
Number of infants with acute care visits	29	36
Number of acute care visits	163	186
Number of infants with failure to thrive	0	1
Number of infants reported abused	2	4
Number of infants in foster care	0	2

[a]The difference in the two means is statistically significant ($p < 0.05$).

physically abused and required foster care. One infant in the early-discharge group died of sudden infant death syndrome during the first year of follow-up. There were no deaths in the control group.

There were no statistically significant differences between the groups in the developmental quotient of infants as measured by the Bayley scale of infant development. Two infants, one in each group, had developmental quotients below 80. Seven infants (four in the early-discharge group and three in the control group) were at or below the fifth percentile in physical growth (weight and length) at the end of the follow-up period. Of these seven infants, one was a twin and two had been small for gestational age at birth. These three infants were in the experimental group.

Despite the nurse's maintaining frequent telephone contact with the parents in the early-discharge group, according to the study protocol, parents initiated more than 300 telephone calls to the nurse during the follow-up period. Seventy-four percent of the calls were made within the first six months after discharge. Parents' concerns were classified into five major areas and ranked according to frequency. The five areas were newborn health problems (30 percent), concerns about routine care of the newborn (25 percent), giving information (22 percent), requesting information (13 percent), and maternal concerns (10 percent). Newborn health problems included questions regarding apnea monitoring, respiratory infections, gastrointestinal problems, fevers, hernias, medicines, skin rashes, injuries, ear infections, and nonspecific symptoms. Concerns about routine newborn care included questions or problems with feeding, elimination, hearing, sleep, hygiene, immunization, and development. Giving information included reports by the parents of the infant's condition, providing new telephone numbers for parents, and canceling or making appointments for home visits by the nurse or for the follow-up clinic. Requests for information included questions about tests and equipment, requests for physicians' telephone numbers and referrals to community agencies and parent support groups. Maternal concerns included questions about the resumption of sexual activities, frustrations about living conditions, scheduling clinic appointments, and problems with monitor companies. The number and type of telephone calls initiated by parents did not differ according to the type of medical insurance held by the parents.

Total charges for the initial hospitalizations for the 79 infants were $4,974,710, consisting of $4,450,910 in hospital charges and $523,800 for physicians' fees (Table 3). The average hospital charge was $56,341 and the average physician's charge was $6,803 for each infant. The difference in the mean hospital charge

TABLE 3
Costs of Care for Very-Low-Birth-Weight Infants

	Early-Discharge Group	Control Group
Charges for initial hospitalization		
Number of infants	39	40
Total	$1,853,297	$2,597,613
Mean	47,520[a]	64,940[a]
Range	21,729–106,409	23,619–131,882
SD	19,856	31,545
Charges for physician's services		
Number of infants	38[b]	39[b]
Total	$225,465	$298,335
Mean	5,933[c]	7,649[c]
Range	2,275–10,625	3,125–15,725
SD	2,164	3,169
Costs related to nurse specialist's services		
Number of families	36	0
Total cost of nurse specialist's time	$19,264	—
Mean cost of nurse specialist's time	535	—
Total telephone charges	966	—
Mean telephone charges	27	—
Total travel costs	500	—
Mean travel costs	14	—

[a]The difference between the two means is statistically significant ($p < 0.01$) by a one-tailed test.

[b]Physician's charge data were unavailable for one infant in each group.

[c]The difference between the two means is statistically significant ($p < 0.01$) by a one-tailed test.

between the early-discharge group ($47,520) and the control group ($64,940) was $17,420; this difference was statistically significant ($p < 0.01$). The difference in the mean physician's charge between the early-discharge group ($5,933) and the control group ($7,649) was $1,716, which was also significant ($p < 0.01$). The mean hospital charge for the early-discharge group was 26.8 percent less than that for the control group. The mean physician's charge was 22.4 percent less than that for the control group. The mean combined hospital and physician's charges for the early-discharge group were $19,136, or 26.4 percent less than for the control group.

The difference between the groups cannot all be counted as savings, since the costs of the nurse specialist's services must be included for the early-discharge group. The parents of the infants discharged early were not charged for the nurse's services, so no charge data exist. Therefore, the actual cost of providing this care was used for this part of the analysis. The cost of the time spent by the nurse in direct care of the infants and families was considered, as well as telephone time, time spent on home visits, travel time to and from home vists, and administrative time. Telephone charges and travel costs were included in the analysis.

The total cost of the home follow-up care for 33 infants for 18 months and 6 infants for 6 months was $20,730 (Table 3). This is a mean cost of $576 per infant and consists of the following: the cost of the time spent by the nurse specialist with families before discharge (a mean of $137 per family), the time spent by the nurse specialist with families after discharge ($398 per family), $27 for telephone calls, and $14 in travel costs for home visits. All the families in the early-discharge group lived within 45 miles (72 km) of the hospital.

DISCUSSION

Programs of early hospital discharge for low-birth-weight infants can potentially decrease iatrogenic illness and hospital-acquired infections, enhance parent-infant interaction, and decrease hospital costs for care. With the introduction of diagnosis-related groups and prospective payment systems, such programs are an econonic necessity. However, such programs are scarce in the United States, and the majority of them have dealt with healthy infants with higher birth weights and greater gestational age than the infants in our study, and most of the infants have been born to middle-class families.[11] Moreover, few of these programs provide the much-needed assistance in caring for the infant during the important transition period in the home, after hospital discharge.

On the basis of our findings, we conclude that early discharge of very-low-birth-weight infants according to the standards used in this study is safe, feasible, and cost-effective and provides continuity of care. The hospital-based approach has several advantages: it provides continuity of care by having a nurse with specialized knowledge and skills in caring for these families and infants provide the direct care; it includes the nurse as an integral part of the hospital staff and community network, with backup available from physicians familiar with the past progress of the infant; and it makes the services of the nurse available to the families seven days a week through a telephone service. The continued home monitoring of the infant's physical status, the parents' ability to cope, their compliance with specialized medical procedures, and their use of any equipment required for high-risk infants discharged early mean that home follow-up care must be provided by nurses who have specialized in high-risk neonatal care. The need for this kind of follow-up care can only increase as smaller infants with many complex health problems survive and as the complexity of their home care increases.

Using the study methods described above, we found that infants in the early-discharge group were able to be discharged 11.2 days earlier than controls (46.5 vs. 57.7 days). These figures compare with nationally reported means of 63 and 57 days of hospitalization for infants with birth weights under 1500 g.[12] The early-discharge group in our study had a mean birth weight of only 1187 g.

The safety of early discharge using this approach is supported by the similar numbers of rehospitalizations and acute care visits for infants in the early-discharge and control groups, which are also comparable to nationally reported figures.[13] Furthermore, there were no infants with failure to thrive because of parental neglect, there was no reported physical abuse of infants, and there were no foster placements among the infants in the early-discharge group who were followed by the nurse specialist. These outcomes were achieved in a sample in which 42 percent of the mothers had less than a high-school education, 69 percent were unmarried, 75 percent were insured by Medicaid, 69 percent had a reported annual income of less than $7,500, 11 percent had no telephone, and 72 percent had to rely on the police or public transportation in an emergency.

In addition to its safety, this type of hospital-based home follow-up care for high-risk infants is feasible and cost-effective. Even with the largely poor, often transient, mothers in the early-discharge group, loss of high-risk infants to medical follow-up was not a problem in this study. Because of the continuity of care provided by the nurse, her ability to handle the problems of high-risk infants and their parents' concerns, and her availability seven days a week, all but one family in the early-discharge group remained in the study until its completion. That one family moved to another part of the country. Moreover, the direct cost of the nurse specialist's services was very low, especially as compared with the charges for hospitalization and physicians' services for these infants. The mean savings in hospital and physician's charges for the early-discharge group totaled $19,136, or 26.4 percent of the average charge for the control group, minus the added cost of the nurse specialist ($576). This yielded a net savings of $18,560 per infant, or 25.6 percent of the charges for the control group.

Since data on actual charges were used for physicians' and hospital fees, whereas data on costs were used to determine the offsetting expenses related to the services provided by the nurse specialist, the costs calculated for the two groups of infants were not fully comparable. However, $576 is only 0.8 percent of the combined mean hospital and physician's fees for the control group. If the nurse services were charged at 50 percent more or even at double their direct cost, they would still constitute only 1.2 percent or 1.6 percent of that amount, respectively. Thus, even if the charge for these services were $1,152 (i.e., $576 × 2), the savings would far outweigh these charges.

These figures should be compared with the hospital and physician charges for the early-discharge group, which were 26.4 percent lower than those for the control group. The results of this study suggest the potential for substantial savings in health care costs if our approach were followed nationwide. If only half the 36,000 very-low-birth-weight infants born in the United States each year were discharged early according to the protocol we tested, the annual savings could be as much as $334 million ($19,136 − $576 × 18,000).

It should be noted that the data on the cost of hospital and physician's care were based on actual charges, not on costs. From the perspective of private insurers and self-paying patients, that is a reasonable approach. However, it may overstate the potential savings to society if charges exceed costs—as they do in some, but not necessarily all, cases. If the hospital and physician's charges were 25 percent, 50 percent, 75 percent, or 100 percent more than the costs of delivering the services, then the potential cost savings from early discharge of half the very-low-birth-weight infants born each year would be $265 million, $219 million, $186 million, or $162 million, respectively. Thus, even estimating conservatively that half the very-low-birth-weight infants could be discharged early and assuming that charges for all items were double the actual costs, the total savings nationwide could be as much as $162 million annually.

Earlier discharge of low-birth-weight infants provides numerous potential benefits. These benefits may be offset, however, if high-risk infants are discharged early, and impse increased and highly stressful responsibilities for monitoring and care on their parents. This is particularly true if the parents lack the benefit of supportive programs and continuous contact with persons who are knowledgeable about and familiar with the problems and care of their infants since birth. A need for this type of support and continuity of care was suggested in our study by the number and types of calls the parents made to the nurse, the number of infants who required home apnea monitoring and medication, the number of families that remained in the study, and subsequently, the number of infants who continued to receive medical follow-up.

As prospective payment systems expand, it may well be financially beneficial for hospitals themselves to institute programs such as the one described here. For a hospital, the value of such a service lies in the improved, extended service it can provide to the families of high-risk infants, especially in view of the demonstrated need for such a program and its usefulness to families. Society also stands to benefit in many ways that cannot be quantified—in the support provided to families through the difficult period after discharge, and the potential reduction in child abuse and foster placement, for example, as well as in reduced health care costs.

ABOUT THE AUTHORS

At the time of writing, Dorothy Brooten, PhD, Savitri Kumar, MD, Linda P. Brown, PhD, Priscilla Butts, MSN, Steven A. Finkler, PhD, Susan Bakewell-Sachs, MSN, Ann Gibbons, MSN, and Maria Delivoria-Papadopoulos, MD, were from the Division of Women's Health and Childbearing, University of Pennsylvania School of Nursing, and the Division of Neonatology, Department of Pediatrics, University of Pennsylvania School of Medicine, Philadelphia.

REFERENCES

1. National Center for Health Statistics, *Monthly Vital Statistics Report, 1975,* Vol. 25, No. 10; *1976,* Vol. 26, No. 12; *1977,* Vol. 27, No. 11; *1978,* Vol. 29, No. 1; *1979,* Vol. 28, No. 13; and *1981,* Vol. 30, No. 12 (Washington, DC: U.S. Department of Health, Education & Welfare, 1976, 1978, 1979, 1980, 1981, and 1982).

2. K.-S. Lee, N. Paneth, L. M. Gartner, M. A. Pearlman, and L. Gruss, "Neonatal Mortality: An Analysis of the Recent Improvement in the United States," *American Journal of Public Health,* 70 (1980), 15-21; and R. Cohen and D. Stevenson, "Prenatal Care for VLBW Infants," *Perinatology & Neonatology,* 7 (1983), 13-16.

3. S. Buckwald, W. A. Zorn, and E. A. Egan, "Mortality and Follow-Up Data for Neonates Weighing 500 to 800 g at Birth," *American Journal of Diseases of Children,* 138 (1984), 779-782; M. C. McCormick, "The Contribution of Low Birth Weight to Infant Mortality and Childhood Morbidity," *New England Journal of Medicine,* 312 (1985), 82-90; and S. Saigal, P. Rosenbaum, B. Stoskopf, and R. Milner, "Follow-Up of Infants 501 to 1,500 gm Birth Weight Delivered to Residents of a Geographically Defined Region with Perinatal Intensive Care Facilities," *Journal of Pediatrics,* 100 (1982), 606-613.

4. A. W. Gottfried, P. Wallace-Lande, S. Sherman-Brown, J. King, C. Coen, and J. E. Hodgman, "Physical and Social Environment of Newborn Infants in Special Care Units," *Science,* 214 (1981), 673-675; F. H. Bess, B. F. Peek, and J. J. Chapman, "Further Observations on Noise Levels in Infant Incubators," *Pediatrics,* 63 (1979), 100-106; and P. Glass, G. B. Avery, K. N. S. Subramanian, M. P. Keys, A. M. Sostek, and D. S. Friendly, "Effect of Bright Light in the Hospital Nursery on the Incidence of Retinopathy of Prematurity," *New England Journal of Medicine,* 313 (1985), 401-404.

5. M. M. Desmond, A. Vorderman, and M. Salinas, "The Family and Premature Infant after Neonatal Intensive Care," *Texas Medicine,* 76(1) (1980), 60-63; J. Hayes, "Premature Infant Development: The Relationship of Neonatal Stimulation, Birth Condition and Home Environment," *Pediatric Nursing,* 6(November-December 1980), 33-36; J. A. Jeffcoate, M. E. Humphrey, and J. K. Lloyd, "Disturbance in Parent-Child Relationship Following Preterm Delivery," *Developmental Medicine and Child Neurology,* 21 (1979), 344-352; and C. P. Larson, "Efficacy of Prenatal and Postpartum Home Visits on Child Health and Development," *Pediatrics,* 66 (1980), 191-197.

6. S. A. Schroeder, J. A. Showstack, and H. E. Roberts, "Frequency and Clinical Description of High-Cost Patients in 17 Acute-Care Hospitals," *New England Journal of Medicine,* 300 (1979), 1306-1309; and S. L. Kaufman and D. S. Shepard, "Costs of Neonatal Intensive Care by Day of Stay," *Inquiry,* 19 (1982), 167-178.

7. D.-J. B. Walker, A. Feldman, B. R. Vohr, and W. Oh, "Cost-Benefit Analysis of Neonatal Intensive Care for Infants Weighing Less than 1,000 grams at Birth," *Pediatrics,* 74 (1984), 20-25.

8. H. Hurt, "Continuing Care of the High-Risk Infant," *Clinics in Perinatology,* 11 (1984), 3-17.

9. McCormick, "The Contribution of Low Birth Weight to Infant Mortality and Childhood Morbidity."

10. National Center for Health Statistics, *Factors Associated with Low Birthweight,* DHEW Pub. No. (PHS) 80-1915 (Washington, DC: Department of Health, Education & Welfare, 1980).

11. C. H. Bauer and W. Tinklepaugh, "Low Birth Weight Babies in the Hospital: A Survey of Recent Changes in Their Care, with Special Emphasis on Early Discharge," *Clinical Pediatrics,* 10 (1971), 467-469; R. B. Berg and A. J. Salisbury, "Discharging Infants of Low Birth Weight: Reconsideration of Current Practice," *American Journal of Diseases of Children* 122 (1971), 414-417; H. L. Britton and J. R. Britton, "Efficacy of Early Newborn Discharge in a Middle-Class Population," *American Journal of Diseases of Children,* 138 (1984), 1041-1046; R. G. Dillard and S. B. Korones, "Lower Discharge Weight and Shortened Nursery Stay for Low-Birth-Weight Infants," *New England Journal of Medicine,* 288 (1973), 131-133; and H. Hurt, L. Gealt, M. Johnson, M. Wurtz, and N. Brodsky, "Home Visiting Nurses Are Beneficial in Care of Intensive Care Nursery Graduates," *Pediatric Research,* 19(4, part 2) (1985), 239 A, abstract.

12. McCormick, "The Contribution of Low Birth Weight to Infant Mortality and Childhood Morbidity"; and M. Hack, D. DeMonterice, I. R. Merkatz, P. Jones, and A. A. Fanaroff, "Rehospitalization of the Very-Low-Birth-Weight Infant: A Continuum of Perinatal and Environmental Morbidity," *American Journal of Diseases of Children,* 135 (1981), 263-265.

13. Hack et al., "Rehospitalization of the Very-Low-Birth-Weight Infant"; and M. C. McCormick, S. Shapiro, and B. H. Starfield, "Rehospitalization in the First Year of Life for High-Risk Survivors," *Pediatrics,* 66 (1980), 991-999.

Part 3

THE RECORD AS A DATA SOURCE

Measuring Utilization and Impact of Home Care Services: A Systems Model Approach for Cost-Effectiveness

Suzanne Rie Day

INTRODUCTION

Policy Objectives

Voices of experience have invited attention to the desired objectives of long-term care.[1] However, after a decade of demonstrations of alternative community-based programs, an Urban Institute review seeking policy implications found it difficult to make meaningful comparisons; program objectives had been diverse, case-mix and services quite varied.[2]

Neither system objectives, nor criteria for measuring progress toward ob-

Reprinted with permission from *Home Health Care Services Quarterly,* 5 (Summer 1984), pp. 5–23, copyright © 1984, The Haworth Press.

This research was partially supported by a research grant DHEW, HCFA 18-P-97362/501 and a dissertation grant, 90-AT-2019/01, from the Administration on Aging. An earlier version of this paper was presented at the 110th Annual Meeting of the American Public Health Association, November 16, 1982. Montreal, Canada.

jectives, are addressed sufficiently in public policy debate and analytic literature on the several types of services which compose what is known as long-term care. When criteria *are* discussed, they are usually those by which to assess quality of care.[3] Standards for quality of service are useful objectives *within programs,* but for planning and public financing a long-term care system, objectives need to be in terms of relationships *between parts* of that system. We need information on the flow of utilization between types of long-term care providers.

Our society's stated goals for long-term care are not consistent with one another.[4] We want quality, accessibility, and affordability. "Cost containment" is the political objective heard regularly even while the numbers at risk of needing chronic care are growing. Although politically attractive, the words "cost containment" mask the complexity of comparing programs for their cost-effectiveness. Unlike cost-benefit comparisons, where inputs and outcomes are both measured in dollars, cost-effectiveness ratios are calculated by dollars used per increment of change toward a specific objective.[5] No matter what objectives are declared, measuring movement toward a goal involves (1) initial assessment (entry characteristics), (2) accounting of program use (resources absorbed), and (3) outcome measures related to the objectives. Goals for the long-term care system are unspecified, standard measures for entry and exit condition are still emergent, and resources used vary widely across programs.

Meanwhile, researchers have sought to shed light on the dim area of cost-effectiveness even without defining objectives. Some have presumed community-based alternatives should meet the same needs for care as nursing homes, and proceeded to compare costs for these "equal products."[6] Some have differentiated expected outcome, e.g., rehabilitation, terminal care, maintenance of function, to distinguish utilization patterns, but norms have not been suggested by which to evaluate progress toward an objective.[7]

Political attention to cost-effectiveness of alternative forms of long-term care has focused almost completely on specification of costs, with efforts to project future costs. However, unless a relationship is established between costs and effects, expenditures can neither be evaluated nor compared across programs. This paper explores a systems model, seeking to link the costs of home care to types of users and their situation at discharge from home care service.

Although preventing and postponing entry to nursing home seems a political objective for community care, only one study, by Kraus and Armstrong, has been found which directly separated home care users by the impact services at home had on their propensity to enter residential institutions.[8] Many home service demonstrations have compared those who enrolled with a control group for differences in mental functioning, mortality rate, performance of functional tasks.[9] These differences, however, do not translate into program designs for meeting political objectives. Although there is not clear consensus, political objectives are less directed toward improving mental function or extending longevity of patients than toward reducing the escalation of costs for medical and maintenance care.

Service Use in Systems Model

Older adults' use of home care services is within a context of prior conditions and follow-up needs. Viewing home care as a system within a larger system, the entry, service use, and exit characteristics can be seen as input-throughput-output questions:

Who enters formal home care services, and at what levels of need?

What services do they use, and for what periods of time?

Why do they discontinue home care, and with what need for services?

Figure 1 illustrates a conceptual model of home care as one type of service within an environment of preexisting and subsequent conditions. The model assumes: (1) that those who receive home services do so with a variety of personal and contextual characteristics; (2) that care may be from a variety of helpers, intermittent or continuous, and of varied frequency and duration; and (3) that users of formal home care may cease to use services because they no longer need assistance, because other services—in the community or from an institution—match their needs better, or because they die. (The entire topic of death is usually missing from discussion of objectives for long-term care.)

The empirical study which follows uses records of one agency to examine the "interior" of this model. As a case study, the findings are descriptive of one population, not prescriptive for policy or administration of programs. Numerous other populations might be analyzed with the same model, moving toward identifying norms for various types of community care, and building toward identification of the transfers across the network of services as in a Markov process.

Hypotheses were explored anticipating relationships between clients' entry characteristics, patterns of use of home services, and their need for services at time of discharge:

1. Utilization of care would be more a function of previous level of care, referral source, type of payment (contextual variables), than of living arrangement, age, or sex (personal characteristics).

2. Intensity of service would be positively associated with likelihood of discharge to self-care, at least for the cases of relatively short duration.

The objective for the geriatric home care program was defined as prevention

FIGURE 1
Indicators for Analyzing Geriatric Home Care System

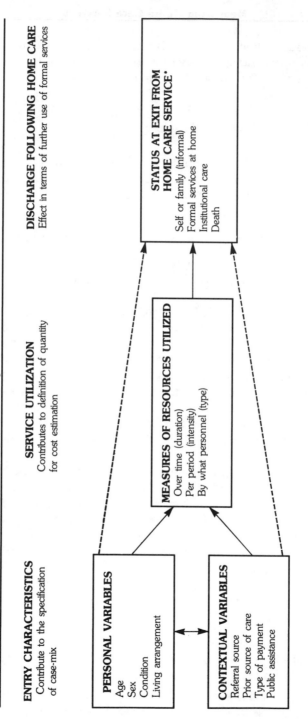

ENTRY CHARACTERISTICS
Contribute to the specification of case-mix

SERVICE UTILIZATION
Contributes to definition of quantity for cost estimation

DISCHARGE FOLLOWING HOME CARE
Effect in terms of further use of formal services

PERSONAL VARIABLES
Age
Sex
Condition
Living arrangement

CONTEXTUAL VARIABLES
Referral source
Prior source of care
Type of payment
Public assistance

MEASURES OF RESOURCES UTILIZED
Over time (duration)
Per period (intensity)
By what personnel (type)

STATUS AT EXIT FROM HOME CARE SERVICE*
Self or family (informal)
Formal services at home
Institutional care
Death

*Some who exit home care later return; these interruptions are not "exits" from records, but inactive service periods.

or postponement of entry to nursing home. Outcome status was noted in terms of care subsequent to home service. The costs of the program were considered in terms of the resources used; skill level of personnel and visits per week (intensity); and length of service (duration in months or years).

METHODOLOGY

Data

The questions raised above—Who comes into home care? What services do they use? How do they leave?—had to be addressed with records of home care users which were thorough in their documentation, numerous enough for the level of disaggregation called for in the model, and longitudinally complete from entry through exit so that post-home-service needs for care could be calculated, and full service utilization could be included. Only a few data sets in the United States seemed to fit the purpose of the study, and only one was found publicly accessible. The dearth of adequate data on non-facility-based health care utilization is a serious methodological obstacle to cost-effectiveness analysis.

San Francisco Home Health Service, Inc. (SFHHS), is a metropolitan agency emphasizing continuity of care and home aide service. By contract with DHEW[10] the case records spanning 18 years (1957-1975) were prepared for computer analysis by retrospectively coding client information from admissions interview, and documenting service history from the monthly billing, nursing, and administrative reports. For the present study, cases were screened to meet the following criteria: age 65 or older at admission, entering on or after 1/1968 and before 1/1975, and not Kaiser contract cases, which were specifically only paraprofessional services. The resulting set of 2,436 records was not a sample, but the universe of case records of SFHHS which fit the criteria above.[11]

Discussion of Data

Although the computer-readable records were thorough, gaps in information occur with retrospective studies. Examples of omissions and problems:

- Records had been maintained for billing purposes; therefore services provided by others (not SFHHS) or for which no source of payment was billed, would not have been documented; this could affect analysis of service intensity.
- Records were kept on a monthly basis, with no indication of how many days in that month a person received care; this could distort analysis of length of stay.

- Records held some functional assessment information, primarily recorded as what the agency could do for the client; only proxy indicators were available for estimating client condition; for most cases no information was available on function.
- Records on sociodemographic characteristics at entry were thorough, but long-term cases need periodic reassessment of situation, e.g., living arrangement.

There are very strong advantages of these data as examples of the home care population even after acknowledging the handicaps. This was not an experiment or demonstration, but an ongoing program where factors affecting utilization can be analyzed as a "natural history." The clients had continuity of care, whether continuous or with interruptions, from the full spectrum of home care: aides, social and fieldworkers, therapists, nurses. The level of detail and longitudinal quality of these records appeared to fit the objective of testing the methodology of a systems model with actual case records.

Variables and Analysis Plan

Following the model shown in Figure 1, variables were derived from the intake and history records of SFHHS. Some of the variables were regrouped, derived, combined to match the purposes of this study.[12]

Entry Characteristics. A major problem in planning and analyzing home health services has been the development of criteria for specification of case mix. The identification of subgroups whose service histories differ systematically from others was sought by multivariate analysis of the SFHHS records to deduce case mix.

Variables indicating the personal situation of client at entry were: age, sex, whether living alone or not, and whether or not a nurse visit was recorded with first month's service. Contextual variables were: whether prior care had been at home or in hospital or nursing home, whether or not referral was from a medical source, whether or not the client received public assistance, and what source of payment was expected. (Other details such as diagnosis, year of entry, and marital status were noted but not used in subsequent analyses due to missing data or lack of directionality. Functional assessment ratings were not available for most of these retrospectively coded case records.)

These categorial characteristics were described using one- and two-way distributions. Personal and contextual characteristics were first examined for associations within their own classification, then for relationships between personal and contextual characteristics. Strength of association among the entry characteristics is summarized by the Percent Reduction in Error (PRE) for each pair, as described below. Strongly associated characteristics help in interpreting the types of clients discussed following multivariate analyses.

Utilization: Duration and Intensity. Since 20 percent of the cases had interruptions of a month or more in their service history, duration was measured both by months elapsed between entry and discharge, and by months with services from SFHHS. Intensity variables included actual number of visits from each type of provider, proportion of total visits which were nurse visits, and average of all visits per month.

Exit Status. Information in the SFHHS records on "closing reason" and "closing plan" was cross-tabulated and categorized as: died, entered hospital or nursing institution, discharged to self-care or informal care, or expected to continue receiving some type of formal care while living at home. Exit situation was established for 84 percent of the cases—8 percent were still active cases at close of data collection, and 8 percent had incomplete records.

Multivariate Analysis

Employing the SEARCH program,[13] the categorical entry characteristics were sorted for their usefulness in predicting variance in duration and intensity of home services. Identified "types" of utilizers were then compared for exit status by contingency table analysis.

FINDINGS IN CASE HISTORIES

Who Entered Home Care?

The profile of the geriatric cases entering SFHHS is indicated by the one-way distributions of entry characteristics:

Age: Mean (and median) 77; 45 percent were in 70's.

Sex: 30 percent were men, both above and below median age.

Living alone: 64 percent (including half the men).

Living with spouse only: 21 percent.

Living with others: 15 percent.

Use of nurse: 73 percent had nurse visit recorded first month (less likely for those living alone than for those with others).

Those were considered the personal characteristics, while the following were the contextual variables surrounding the older person:

Prior locus of care: 49 percent hospital or nursing home, 51 percent at home.

Referral source: 43 percent health or medical, 57 percent other.

Public assistance recipient: 54 percent no, 46 percent yes.

Pay plan at entry: 33 percent Medicare, 42 percent state (or county), 25 percent not-public.

Bivariate distributions showed no significant relationships among the personal characteristics, weak associations between personal and contextual characteristics, and very strongly linked contextual variables.

When the number of cases is so large, significant chi-squares may be found without the association having useful importance for predicting where a case would fall on one variable given knowledge of its position on another. Figure 2 indicates with arrowheads the Percent Reduction in Error (PRE, the Goodman-Kruskal Lambda)[14] in estimating the client's level on that variable when the level is known for the variable at the foot of the arrow. For example, knowledge of pay plan can reduce error in estimating whether or not a client is on public assistance by 73 percent; knowing status on public assistance only reduces error in estimating pay plan by 38 percent. (A person on state pay plan is almost always on public assistance, but public assistance clients enter home care under a variety of payment plans.)

What Services Were Used and for How Long?

Figure 3 summarizes the findings for the multivariate SEARCH for entry characteristics useful for predicting duration of home care: Pay plan was the most powerful predictor both of mean number of months served and of months elapsed between entry and discharge. Clients with payment from state sources averaged five months longer than those with payment from Medicare and not-public sources—13.4 and 8.7 months respectively.

The clients with state pay plans who had been in hospital before home care averaged close to 15 months, those who had not, 11 months. (At this point the program stopped running since no other split could account for 0.5 percent of the variance—see note 13.)

Figure 4 shows the more detailed branching of the SEARCH program using intensity measure of percentage of visits by nurse as the dependent variable. While the overall mean was 20 percent nursing in these case records, state-pay clients averaged 12 percent while Medicare and not-public cases averaged 26 percent. The latter subdivided into categories by whether or not the client lived alone; clients living alone used lower proportion of nursing than those living with other(s). Most state clients lived alone, but that did not divide the group on its quite low use of nurse visits.

From the combination of these findings on duration and intensity patterns, the impact of pay plan on utilization is sharply divided; the strongest predictor of long duration (state pay) predicts low levels of nursing intensity and vice versa (Medicare and not-public pay plans).

FIGURE 2
Percent Reduction in Error of Estimating a Characteristic Given Information on the Distribution of Another Variable (Goodman-Kruskal Lambda)*

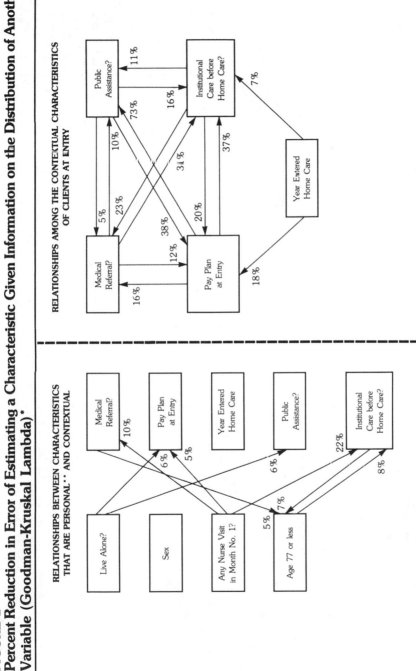

*Relationships which indicate a percent reduction in error of estimate (PRE) lower than 5% were excluded from these diagrams.

**None of the personal/familial variables had Goodman-Kruskal Lambda values as high as 5% when examined in relation to one another.

N = 2436 or slightly fewer on some relationships due to missing data.

FIGURE 3
Multivariate Sort* for Best Predictors of Duration

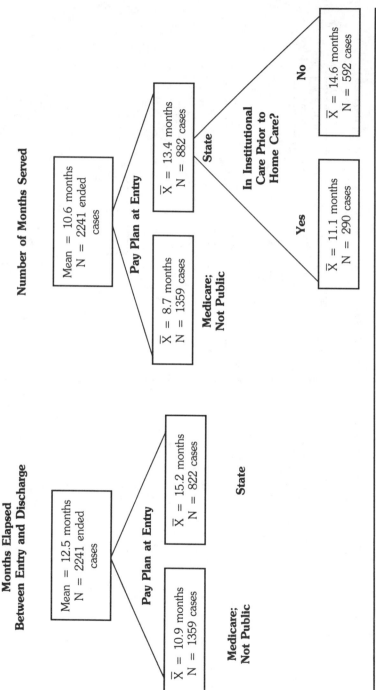

Months Elapsed Between Entry and Discharge

Mean = 12.5 months
N = 2241 ended cases

Pay Plan at Entry

$\overline{X}$ = 10.9 months
N = 1359 cases

Medicare;
Not Public

$\overline{X}$ = 15.2 months
N = 822 cases

State

Number of Months Served

Mean = 10.6 months
N = 2241 ended cases

Pay Plan at Entry

$\overline{X}$ = 8.7 months
N = 1359 cases

Medicare;
Not Public

$\overline{X}$ = 13.4 months
N = 882 cases

State

In Institutional Care Prior to Home Care?

Yes

$\overline{X}$ = 11.1 months
N = 290 cases

No

$\overline{X}$ = 14.6 months
N = 592 cases

*ISR: OSIRIS-IV SEARCH Program—Variables entered in each run of the SEARCH program were: whether living alone; sex; age; whether nursing was recorded in first month; whether on public assistance; pay plan; prior locus of care; whether medically referred.

FIGURE 4
Best Predictors* of the Proportion of Total Visits Which Were Nursing Visits

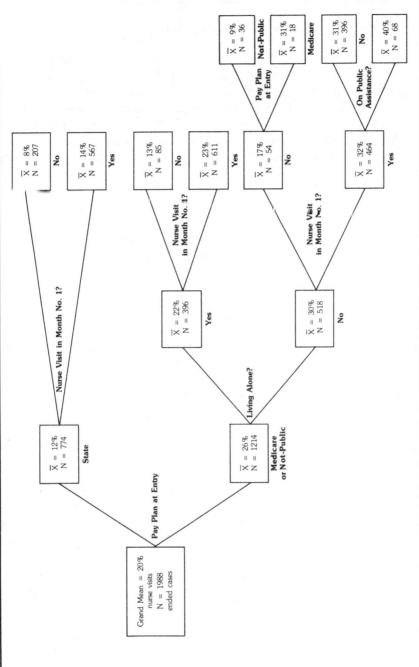

*ISR: OSIRIS-IV SEARCH Program—Variables entered in each run of the SEARCH Program were: whether living alone; sex; age; whether nursing was recorded in first month; whether on public assistance; pay plan; prior locus of care; whether medically referred.

Why Did Cases Terminate Home Service?

One-third of all cases were discharged to self-care or to care informally arranged. Another third left to enter institutional care, either hospital or nursing home. Formal care in the community was anticipated in the closing plans of about a fifth, and fewer than one-fifth died. (This distribution is shown in Table 1.)

Those whose discharge was to self or informal care were significantly younger (75.4 years) than the mean, likely to have come from hospital (2/3), to have been medically referred, and to have Medicare Part A coverage at outset of home care. Almost three-fourths of those who left to self or informal care did so with home care service lasting under six months, and the average intensity of care was 10 percent higher for cases served six months or less compared to others of any exit status. Those who entered from hospital were more likely to leave home care to self or family care than for any other reason.

TABLE 1

Mean and (Median) Elapsed Months of Service by Exit Status and Pay Plan (N = 1,974)

Pay Plan at Entry	Exit Status of Discharged Cases			
	Informal, Self, Family 31% N = 614	Formal Care at Home 20% N = 399	Institution (about 1/3 not hospitalized, 2/3 hospitalized) N = 633	Died 17% N = 328
State funding, special (100% on public assistance. None receiving nurse visit in month No. 1.) 13% N = 253	9 (4) N = 61	18 (9) N = 63	20 (10) N = 88	18 (13) N = 41
State funding (Used nurse in month No. 1.) 27% N = 533	12 (6) N = 129	15 (10) N = 100	17 (8) N = 203	19 (12) N = 101
Medicare A or B 35% N = 695	8 (4) N = 254	12 (7) N = 137	15 (6) N = 194	11 (5) N = 110
Other pay plan 25% N = 493	7 (2) N = 170	11 (5) N = 99	12 (6) N = 148	17 (9) N = 76

Cases leaving for hospital or nursing home care were significantly older (78.9 years) than others. Their average duration of home service was longer than those discharged to community settings; those who died while receiving home services also had long duration of care. Otherwise, those who died were distinguished by a higher proportion of men than expected (1/2), and a far lower proportion living alone. Formal care in the community was a broadly inclusive category, not distinguished by entry characteristics. The pay plan types can now be combined with exit types; it is this linking of utilization pattern and exit status which seems critical for examining resources used.

Contingency Table Analysis of Entry Types by Exit Status

When pay plan at entry and status at discharge are examined in cross-tabulation in Table 1, the duration of those who left to informal care is seen to be from 3 to 9 months lower than the average length of service for other exits, regardless of pay plan. Note that the median months of service were half the mean in many categories, suggesting the impact of those few who were maintained on service for years. Intensity of service is seen in Figure 5 to decline steadily by pay plan from Medicare, through not-public, to state regardless of exit status. Note that "Title XX"[15] state cases were those showing no nursing at first month, representing a very low intensity of nursing visits and long duration.

Change of pay plan from Medicare at entry to state or not-public was not included in the design of the present study. Knowledge of Medicare would suggest the long-term clients who entered on Medicare might have shifted to another source of payment. Nevertheless, the chances of a state client leaving to informal care were only one-half as great as the chances of informal exit by a Medicare client. The chances of a Medicare client leaving to institutional care were less than three-fourths those of a state-pay client.

DISCUSSION

Case Study Results

Disaggregating case-mix deductively from patterns of service use yielded distinct types corresponding to the post-acute, restorative clients on Medicare and the chronic, maintenance clients who were likely to have a state pay plan. (Those whose pay plan was not public held an intermediate, more complex position.) These client types appear distinct from utilization and exit patterns even in the absence of functional assessment measures. The outcomes for the younger, post-hospital Medicare client who lives with spouse would

FIGURE 5
Mean Intensity of Service for Exit-by-Pay-Plan Groups

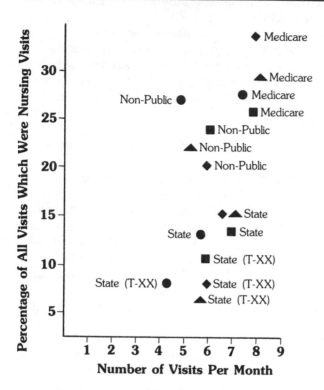

Exit Status
- ● Informal setting or self-care
- ▲ Formal community
- ◆ Formal institution
- ■ Died

be expected to differ from those of a low-income, older, less medically involved client who lives alone. The state-funded clients averaged over a year
of service with less than two visits per week; fewer than half remained in
the community at discharge, and a few remained on active status at close
of study. Medicare clients were more likely to return to self or informal care
than to any other status at discharge, with service history of two or more
visits a week over periods averaging less than a year.

The first hypothesis, that utilization would be more a function of contextual than of personal variables was supported by the dominance of pay plan
as the entry characteristic most clearly separating duration of cases into the
chronic and acute or post-acute. Utilization appeared in distinct patterns for

the entry pay plan types, but the personal variable of living arrangement was also important to predicting the proportion of home aide and nursing visits. The findings indicate those who live with others use fewer aide services. However, the important personal characteristics of physical and mental status were unavailable, and the proxy of nurse visit recorded in first month was inadequate for assessing condition.

The second hypothesis, that higher intensity of care would be associated with higher likelihood of discharge to self-care, at least for short-term cases, was supported by the duration and intensity of services used by Medicare clients. Frequency distributions showed higher-than-expected intensity of care for those whose discharge was to informal or self-care; other categories of exit did not differ from expected on intensity. There is no suggestion here of a causal relationship between intensity and exit condition, entry condition may be far more influential on outcome than treatment.

These findings from a single agency cannot be used in Markov process analyses of long-term care system exchanges to and from home care. However, finding that as many were discharged to self or family as to institutional care should promote greater attention to the preventive impact formal home services may be making on the demand for nursing home beds.

Methodological Implications

Although the analysis of records from one agency cannot be generalized, the *methods* of addressing the pragmatic questions may prove useful to other studies. Here the longitudinal quality of the case records was utilized only in summary fashion: how long was a full term of home care, how many visits per month were used averaged across the history of service? More trend analysis could be addressed through these or similar data. Combining the intensity variables displayed in Figure 5 with the duration shown in Table 1, distinguishing type, intensity, and duration of service[16] can be seen essential to measuring home care. Studies which have used total visits to measure utilization may have compounded duration effect with intensity effects particularly in assessing long-term care. Regressing number of months served (duration) and visits-per-month (intensity) on total number of visits indicated over 75 percent of the variance in total visits was accounted for by number of months served for every pay plan. Visits-per-month accounted for only 20 percent of the variance in total visits for state and non-public clients, and 10 percent for those on Medicare.

Policy and Policy Research Implications

The distribution of intensity illustrates (Figure 5) how proportion of nurse visits varied more than visits per month. Very likely, agency policy[17] was more flexible on type of staff than on number of staff contacts with client per month. Note the very low number of visits per month, similar to findings in the Minnesota study of Anderson et al.[18]

The concern with costs is, at root, a concern with service utilization; it is the quantity consumed times the price of various types of services which result in cost. Beyond estimating costs of possible future services, policy deliberations continue on which costs should be carried or subsidized with public funds, and which types of "need" should be addressed by which components of a service system. Since some political concern has been expressed over utilization of home services possibly continuing indefinitely, the finding that home service discharges show high proportions returning to independence should provoke interest in the relationship among components of the service system.

For meaningful cost-effectiveness analysis, the uses of service need to be interpreted in the light of the post-service condition of clients. Only by observing such indicators of "outcome" can value of program resources be weighed and ranked for their impact on policy objectives.

Although the records analyzed in this study left lacunae, the relationships identified appear relevant to policy questions. By implication, much of the rhetoric surrounding long-term care alternatives implies the goal is restoration to "maximum levels of functional ability." For assessing alternatives, however, chronic care must be distinguished from acute and curative intervention.[19] Preventing and postponing unnecessary or inappropriate institutional care is broadly implied as a policy objective, yet few reports on alternatives to institutional services actually follow their cases through to subsequent care, independence, or death.

The eventuality of death has not been publicly acceptable for discussion, even within the context of long-term geriatric care policy. Methods of evaluating long-term care, however, must acknowledge mortality as one legitimate outcome. The model of the home care system used for this analysis is proposed as a means to evaluate program effects while applying statistical controls for client type, and measuring resource use across time.

It would be useful to compare other home care service agency records with those of SFHHS. A service utilization study seeking to establish relationships between client condition, use, and outcome needs full information on each level. Home care agencies do not normally keep records with thorough detail on services received by, or available to, clients from other formal providers. Such "external" services simultaneous with or intermittent between spells of home care service could confound the results of examining relationships derived solely from one agency's records. Further, assessing effects of long-term care requires detail on the career of clients following use of agency services. The systems approach presses for longitudinal and thorough specification of client characteristics, resources used, and subsequent service needs.

Hence, prospective panel studies which follow representative samples of older adults through their full complement of informal and formal, inpatient and outpatient service utilization would be far more informative than the retrospective analysis of SFHHS records, or those of any other specific agency.

The idiosyncrasies of chronic disability and geriatric care arrangements, and the political environment surrounding change in delivery of care all contribute to both the *desire* for empirical cost-effectiveness relationships and the *persistent uncertainty* of those relationships. In the British National Health Service, where data would be attainable, Home Helps are presumed so basic to geriatric services that their cost-effectiveness is not rigorously debated; in the United States we ponder the means to bring rational planning to the decision process, normally ignoring the costs and effects of the current arrangements.

ABOUT THE AUTHOR

At the time of writing, Suzanne Rie Day, MA, MPH, PhD, was a research and services development consultant, Egg Harbor, New Jersey.

REFERENCES

1. J. J. Callahan, "How Much, for What, and for Whom?" *American Journal of Public Health,* 71(9) (1981), 987–988; B. D. Dunlop, "Expanded Home-Based Care for the Impaired Elderly: Solution or Pipe Dream?" *American Journal of Public Health,* 70 (1980), 514–519; J. Lavor and M. Callender, "Home Health Cost-Effectiveness: What Are We Measuring?" *Medical Care,* 14 (1976), 866–872; and R. Morris, "Designing Care for the Long-Term Patient: How Much Change is Necessary in the Pattern of Health Provision?" *American Journal of Public Health,* 70(5) (1980), 471–472.

2. M. Stassen and J. Holahan, *Long-Term Care Demonstration Projects: A Review of Recent Evaluations,* working paper P-1227-2 (Washington, DC: Urban Institute, 1981).

3. Callahan, "How Much, for What, and for Whom?"; F. Caro, *Objectives in Long Term Care* (New York: Institute for Social Welfare Research, 1980); and R. L. Kane and R. A. Kane, eds., *Values and Long-Term Care* (Lexington, MA: Lexington Books, 1982).

4. R. L. Kane and R. A. Kane, "The Extent and Nature of Public Responsibility for Long-Term Care," in J. Melzer, F. Farrow, and H. Richman, eds., *Policy Options in Long-Term Care* (Chicago: The University of Chicago Press, 1981), chap. 3.

5. R. N. Grosse, "Cost-Benefit Analysis of Health Service, *The Annals,* 399 (1972), 89–99; Office of Technology Assessment, *The Implications of Cost-Effectiveness Analysis of Medical Technology* (Washington, DC: U.S. Congress, 1980); and A. Williams, "The Cost-Benefit Approach," *British Medical Bulletin,* 30(3) (1974), 252–256.

6. J. Hammond, "Home Health Care Cost Effectiveness: An Overview of the Literature," *Public Health Reports,* 94(4), 1979, 305–311.

7. B. Hicks, J. Segal, and N. Doherty, "The Triage Experiment in Coordinated Care for the Elderly," *American Journal of Public Health,* 71(9) (1981), 991–1003; S. Katz, J. Papsidero, M. H. Kroger, and C. A. Akpom, eds., *Community Care of the Aged: Chronic Disease Service Module* (Lansing: Michigan State University Health Services Education and Research, 1977); B. T. Kurowski, R. E. Schlenker, and G. Tricarico, *Applied Research in Home Health Services, Vol. II: Cost per Episode* (Denver: University of Colorado Medical Center, 1979); and Office of Technology Assessment, *The Implications of Cost-Effectiveness Analysis of Medical Technology.*

8. A. S. Kraus and M. I. Armstrong, "Effect of Chronic Home Care on Admission to Institutions," *Canadian Medical Association Journal,* 117 (1977), 747–749.

9. Hicks, Segal, and Doherty, "The Triage Experiment in Coordinated Care for the Elderly"; F. Skellie, G. M. Mobley, and R. E. Coan, "Cost-Effectiveness of Community-Based Long-Term Care: Current Findings of Georgia's Alternative Health Services Project," *American Journal of Public Health,* 72(4) (1982), 353–358; and W. G. Weissert, T. T. H. Wan, and B. B. Livieratos, *Effects and Costs of Day Care and Homemaker Services for the Chronically Ill: A Randomized Experiment* (Washington, DC: National Center for Health Services Research, Department of Health, Education & Welfare, 1979).

10. The original research grant was to the School of Public Health at University of California at Berkeley; subsequent contract from Office of the Assistant Secretary for Planning and Evaluation, Department of Health, Education, and Welfare, HEW-100-77-0065 to San Francisco Home Health Services, Inc.

11. S. R. Day, *Geriatric Home Care Utilization: San Francisco, 1968-75* (Ann Arbor, MI: Inter-university Consortium for Political and Social Research, 1982).

12. Ibid.

13. The SEARCH program is available in ISR:OSIRIS. IV, a combination of previous AID and THAID programs. A series of dichotomous splits of a "parent" group is examined, and the binary division (split) is made on the "child" group which maximally improves the explained variation of the dependent (parent) group. Interaction detection is facilitated by the table of means of every level of every predictor variable of each group identified. See Sonquist, Baker, and Morgan, *Searching for Structure* (Ann Arbor, MI: Institute for Social Research, 1973). Options in the program were set as follows: mean of each dependent variable was selected as the criterion for seeking the best split; minimum number of cases per group was set at 15, maximum number of groups at 20. Neither of these limits was met before the splits stopped at limit of predicting at least 0.5 percent of the variation. Predictor variables submitted for analysis were personal and contextual as follows: sex; age (less than or equal to 77, over 77); living alone or with others; nurse visit in month number 1; entering from prior institutional care; having medical referral; having state, federal, or non-public pay plan at entry.

14. *Elementary Statistics Using MIDAS* (2nd ed.; Ann Arbor: Statistical Research Laboratory, University of Michigan, 1976), 194–195.

15. "Title XX" is used symbolically here for chore-type and homemaker service. Early years of these case records preceeded Title XX's amendment of the Social Security Act. The State of California carefully regulated Medicaid (Medi-Cal) and Title XX (Adult Services) funds to achieve advantageous federal matching funds. Clients

entered under Division of Social Service funds in far greater numbers than under Medicaid and under Medicare Part A in greater numbers than Part B.

16. N. Robinson, E. Shinn, E. Adam, and F. Moore, *Cost of Homemaker-Home Health Aide and Alternative Forms of Service: A Survey of the Literature* (New York: National Council for Homemaker-Home Health Aide Service, Inc., 1974).

17. S. Rosenfeld, "Factors Affecting Home Health Agency Behavior: An Interactionist View," *Home Health Care Services Quarterly,* 2(2) (1981), 50–100.

18. N. N. Anderson, S. K. Patten, and J. N. Greenberg, *A Comparison of Home Care and Nursing Home Care for Older Persons in Minnesota* (Minneapolis: University of Minnesota, 1980).

19. P. G. Weiler, "Cost-Effective Analysis: A Quandary for Geriatric Health Care Systems," *The Gerontologist,* 14(5) (1974), 414–417.

.

Selected Correlates of Job Performance of Community Health Nurses

Beverly L. Koerner

Development of home health care as an alternative to costly institutional care has increased the need for the nursing profession to monitor job performance through quality assurance programs in home health agencies and to identify variables that influence nurses' job performance. Sources of variation in job performance arise out of the attributes nurses bring to the work situation and the characteristics of the work environment.[1] While studies have been conducted on the performance of nurses employed in hospital settings, much remains unknown regarding the contribution of selected variables in explaining the variance of job performance.

REVIEW OF THE LITERATURE

The theoretical framework for this study was derived from systems theory which is useful in examining the interrelatedness of specific organizational and attribute variables to job performance.[2] Ten variables were selected and organized, using Jelinek's model of the patient care system[3] (see Figure 1).

Reprinted with permission from *Nursing Research,* 30 (January-February 1981), pp. 43–48, copyright © 1981, *American Journal of Nursing Company.*

FIGURE 1
Model of the Patient Care System: Variable Relationships

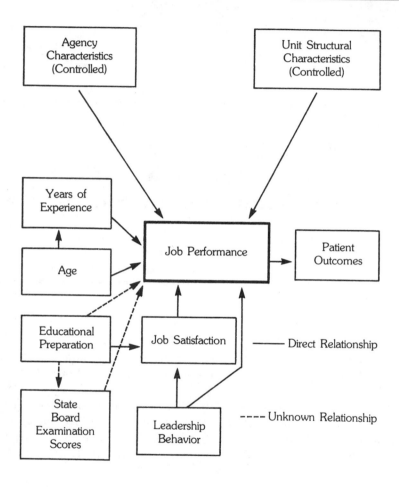

Personnel variables chosen were job satisfaction, years of work experience, age, highest educational preparation attained, and scores on the state board licensure examinations. In the category of agency environment, perceived leadership behavior of the supervisor was selected for a study variable. Extraneous variance as a result of agency size, complexity, and affiliation was controlled by using one agency to procure a sample. Because this agency has two units which are nearly identical in structural characteristics, extraneous variance resulting from staffing ratios, workload, and type of client was also controlled.

The Haussmann et al. (1976) study supports Jelinek's model.[4] The investigators studied five sets of independent variables: contextual variables, unit organizational structure, supervisory staff attitudes and perceptions, unit staff attitudes and perceptions, and nursing staff education. When these five sets (33 variables) were correlated with the dependent variable of job performance of nurses, organizational structure of the hospital unit, leadership style, and job satisfaction were significantly related to job performance.

An extensive review of the literature indicated the following relationships of the independent variables selected for this study with the dependent variable of job performance: negative correlations between biographical information of age and work experience, and job performance; positive correlations between perceived leadership behavior of supervisors and job performance; positive correlatons between job satisfaction and job performance; inconclusive data regarding educational preparation and job performance; and inconclusive data regarding state board scores and job performance.

Dyer, in a study of 200 registered nurses in four Utah hospitals, found that dimensions of job performance could be predicted at significant levels using biographical information such as age and years of work experience.[5] Dyer, Monson, and Van Drimmelen, Dyer et al., and Welches et al., found that age and work experience correlated negatively to job performance.[6]

The relation between supervisory styles and the quality of job performance has received little attention in the nursing literature. Hagen and Wolff, Hegyvary, and Kruse and Stogdill found positive correlations between perceived leadership style of nursing supervisors and job performance of staff.[7] Haussmann et al. found significant differences ($p < .05$) between nurses who received high versus low performance ratings and their perceptions of leader behavior.[8] Highly rated nurses described their supervisors as having strong role assumption, sensitivity, and tolerance.

Herzberg and Slocum et al. concluded that staff morale and productivity are positively correlated.[9] Haussmann et al. found a significant ($p < .05$) positive correlation between job performance and satisfaction as measured by the Job Description Index.[10] In the Welches et al. study, the cluster relating to job satisfaction and opportunity for professional growth differentiated the sample.[11]

The literature revealed contradictory evidence of the relationship between educational preparation and job performance. Significant differences ($p < .05$) among graduating seniors of various programs have been shown in technical skills, leadership, use of the nursing process in structured patient care situations, and communication skills.[12] Nelson found that supervisors of baccalaureate nursing graduates rated their overall competence significantly higher ($p < .05$) than did supervisors of diploma or associate degree graduates.[13] Haussmann et al. and Welches et al. found no significant differences between the educational preparation of nurses and their job performance.[14]

Much research has been done on predicting state board scores from variables related to basic nursing education, but little empirical evidence is available on the relationship between state board scores and job performance. Dubs reported a low, positive correlation ($p < .05$) between state board scores and employers' ratings of job performance for diploma program graduates.[15] Brandt and Metheny attempted to determine if performance as a nurse could be predicted from state board achievement; correlation coefficients for state board scores and supervisors' mean ratings of job performance ranged from $-.14$ for psychiatric nursing to .23 for surgical nursing.[16]

Among studies that examined the relationship between the independent variables, significant, positive correlations were found between job satisfaction and leadership behavior of the supervisor by Haussmann et al. and Pryer and Distefano.[17] Data regarding educational preparation and job satisfaction are inconclusive.[18]

OBJECTIVES AND HYPOTHESES

The objectives of this study were to: (1) assess the relationship between selected attribute and environmental variables and a quantitative rating of job performance of nurses employed in a community health agency and (2) develop a valid and reliable measure of job performance based on the ANA Standards of Nursing Practice.[19] To address the first objective of the study more definitively, two null hypotheses were investigated:

I.   There will be no relationship between scores on the Job Performance Measure and age; work experience; highest educational preparation; state board licensure examination (SBE) scores for medicine, surgery, obstetrics, pediatrics, and psychiatry; job satisfaction; and leader behavior.

II. There will be no relationship between scores on the Job Performance Measure and the largest principal component(s) derived from the 10 independent variables identified in hypothesis I.

METHOD

Definition of Terms

Terms were defined as follows:

> *Job Performance.* The process of giving care, i.e., what the caretaker does.[20] It is operationally defined as total score on the Job Performance Measure developed by the Visiting Nurse Association of Hartford, Inc., and the investigator.

Job Satisfaction. A total score on a five-scale measure of satisfaction, the Job Description Index developed by Smith, Kendall, and Hulin.[21]

Leader Behavior. A total score of respondents on the Consideration and Structure scales of the Leader Behavior Description Questionnaire—Form XII.[22]

Work Experience. Total number of years of work experience in nursing since graduation from a basic educational program in nursing.

Sample

The population consisted of registered nurses, licensed to practice nursing in Connecticut, who were employed by a community health agency, the Visiting Nurse Association of Hartford, Inc. (VNA). The agency met the organizational characteristics identified by Haussmann et al. as a source of variation.[23] The VNA of Hartford has only two units, which are believed to be nearly identical in structural characteristics. Each unit has similar staffing ratios and types of clients, and each uses primary nursing so that every nurse is responsible and accountable for her own case load of clients. Within the two units, staff nurses are responsible to one of six superiors. Complete sets of data were collected from 32 of the 37 nurses who volunteered to participate in the study.

Instruments

Eight instruments were used to measure the independent variables in the study: the Job Description Index (JDI), the Leader Behavior Description Questionnaire—Form XII (LBDQ), the five state board licensure examinations (SBEs), and a biographical data questionnaire. Evidence of content and construct validity data as well as reliability estimates were documented for the instruments. The dependent variable of job performance was measured using the Job Performance Measure (JPM) because existing instruments were inadequate.[24]

The Job Performance Measure. The JPM is a 48-item instrument that can be used by any trained person to rate a nurse's documentation in legal records of the care the nurse gives a client. After an extensive review of the literature, 68 items were written and organized using the ANA standards of quality care as a conceptual framework. Items were reviewed by master's prepared clinicians for clarity and representativeness of five a priori dimensions. Using Thurstone's successive interval scaling method,[25] 48 items with hidden scale weights were selected for inclusion in the final instrument. Situational cues for each item were developed to increase interrater agreement.

A known-groups validity study was conducted, using a sample of 25 nurses at the VNA of Hartford. Six VNA supervisors were asked to identify the 8 most effective and the 8 least effective nurses from the list of 25. An analysis of variance of the mean differences on JPM scores for these two groups of nurses showed a highly significant (p < .01) difference.

An alpha internal consistency reliability coefficient of .81 was generated. A test-retest reliability coefficient of .53 for an average interval of six weeks between ratings was generated for 16 staff nurses at the agency. Interrater agreement for the six supervisors involved in this study was established by having the supervisors independently rate a client record. Additional situational cues were written for two items which failed the 100 percent agreement criterion established.

Data Collection

The six VNA supervisors rated 32 staff nurses' documentation of care given their clients, using the JPM as a record audit tool. Records chosen by the supervisors (for the nurses assigned to their units) reflected clients the nurses were currently visiting and for whom they were primary nurses. No other restrictions were placed on the selection of the records. From January to October 1978 supervisors rated two records for each nurse. The first record was used as the measure of the dependent variable in this study. The second rating was used to measure test-retest reliability. Biographical data, nurses' ratings of supervisors using the LBDQ, and job satisfaction data were collected once, in March 1978, at the VNA.

Statistical Procedures

To examine the first null hypothesis, a multiple regression analysis with a nonhierarchical stepwise solution was used to determine the contributions of each selected independent variable in explaining the variance of the dependent variable. A conventional test of statistical significance (p < .05) was used to determine if the magnitudes of the multiple correlations were statistically significant.

To examine the second null hypothesis, raw scores on the variables were submitted to principal component analysis with Varimax rotation. Only components with eigenvalues greater than or equal to 1.0 were retained. Variables that had a factor loading greater than .40 were used in the naming of that component. The Spearman-Brown prophecy formula was used to estimate the alpha-scale reliabilities of the components. Factor scores for each subject were then entered in a nonhierarchical stepwise multiple regression to determine to what extent the components would explain the variance in the criterion.

RESULTS AND DISCUSSION

Hypothesis I

Means, Ranges, and Standard Deviations of Variables. All variables were treated as continuous except education which was treated as a categorical variable; no assumptions were made concerning directionality of educational preparation. Since only one nurse in the study had completed a master's degree, this category was combined with the generic baccalaureate category. Four nurses had diploma education, five held a diploma with a nongeneric baccalaureate degree, and 23 had a generic baccalaureate in nursing.

Table 1 gives means, ranges, and standard deviations for the other study variables. The range on the JPM was negatively skewed and was restricted. Scores on the LBDQ were compared to data for nine occupational groups on the consideration and structure scales.[26] Mean scores on the consideration dimension ranged from a low of 36.9 for a sample of highway patrol to a high of 42.5 for ministers. The mean score for the six supervisors who

TABLE 1
Descriptive Statistics for the Variables in Hypothesis I[a]

Variables	Range	Maximum Possible Score	$\overline{X}$	S.D.
Job performance	80-100	100	92	5.70
Leadership behavior	44-95	100	76	11.84
Job satisfaction	103-193	216	153	23.49
SBE-Medicine	335-740	800	553	89.39
SBE-Surgery	378-720	800	564	74.15
SBE-Obstetrics	431-708	800	555	68.53
SBE-Pediatrics	350-749	800	560	94.12
SBE-Psychiatry	314-711	800	573	88.15
Work experience	2 months-21 years	—	56 months	55.60
Age	23-50	—	29	6.87

[a]Education, a categorical variable, is omitted.

were rated by the 32 staff nurses in this study was 38.1 On the structure scale, mean scores ranged from a low of 36.6 for aircraft commanders to the highest mean score of 39.7 for highway patrol. The mean score for nurses in this study was 38.3. Nurses' scores on the five scales of the JDI were compared to scale statistics for approximately 635 female employees pooled across 21 industrial plants.[27] The nurses' mean scores on the JDI pay and promotion scales were lower than scale statistics presented for female plant workers. Their satisfaction scores on the work and co-worker scales were higher than the mean of the scale statistics presented. The mean scores on the supervision scale were approximately the same.

Independent Variables Correlation Matrix. Pearson product moment correlation coefficients for the nine independent variables (excluding education) of hypothesis I indicated a significantly ($p < .001$) positive relationship between LBDQ and JDI scores, a highly significant ($p < .001$) positive correlation between age and years of work experience, and a significant correlation between SBE scores (see Table 2 for specific significance levels). Licensure examination scores in surgery and obstetrics were positively ($p < .05$) related to scores on the JDI.

Independent-Dependent Variables Correlation Matrix. Negative correlations were found between age and job performance and between years of work experience and job performance. Younger nurses with less work experience tended to achieve higher scores on the JPM. Younger nurses may be better prepared in recording data because they graduated more recently from a nursing program. Current educational programs emphasize use of the nursing process in caring for clients and recording this process in client records.

Negative correlations were found between perceived leadership of supervisors and job performance and between job satisfaction and job performance. These findings are incongruent with those reported in the literature. SBEs in obstetrics and psychiatry had small, positive relationships with the variable of job performance. The examinations in pediatrics and medicine were correlated negatively with job performance. The only variable to achieve significance was SBE-surgery, which had a moderate, negative correlation ($-.40$, $p < .01$) with job performance.

In general, the negative correlations between the independent variables and job performance may reflect, in part, response variation of nurses in charting their care. For example, although nurses may provide excellent care to clients, other factors such as available time to complete records, ability to write concisely, or the number of clients seen in the day may influence charting of that care. The nursing profession has assumed that record audit is a valid method of measuring the quality of care delivered by the nurse. The tentative findings of this study do not support that assumption.

TABLE 2
Pearson Product-Moment Correlation Coefficients for Variables in Hypothesis I

Variables	Behavior	Job Satisfaction	SBE-Medicine	SBE-Surgery	SBE-Obstetrics	SBE-Pediatrics	SBE-Psychiatry	Work Experience	Age	Job Performance
Leadership behavior										
Job satisfaction	.65[d]									
SBE-Medicine	-.04	.02								
SBE-Surgery	.07	.32[a]	.60[d]							
SBE-Obstetrics	.21	.37[a]	.45[c]	.46[c]						
SBE-Pediatrics	.09	.18	.80[d]	.67[d]	.44[b]					
SBE-Psychiatry	.12	.19	.65[d]	.38[a]	.53[d]	.66[d]				
Work experience	.22	.08	.07	-.05	.09	-.06	-.22			
Age	.23	.06	.06	.01	-.05	.08	-.21	.72[d]		
Job performance	-.19	-.19	-.14	-.40[b]	.04	-.06	.11	-.26	-.23	

[a] $p < .05$.
[b] $p < .01$.
[c] $p < .005$.
[d] $p < .001$.

Multiple Regression Analysis. The purpose of this analysis was to determine the contribution of the 10 selected independent variables to the variance of the dependent variable of job performance. The optimal predictor set was defined as that combination of variables which predicts the criterion with a minimum standard error of estimate.

SBE-surgery had the highest correlation with the criterion and entered the equation on the first step. This variable also had the highest regression weight in the equation. Since the stepwise procedure selects those weights which maximize the multiple correlation, positive or negative, this variable was useful in explaining the variance in job performance. For this step, the multiple correlation achieved significance at $p = .05$. The b weight for surgery achieved significance at $p = .01$ (see Table 3). After the entry of the leader behavior variable in the fifth step, the standard error of estimate began to increase. The variables of job satisfaction, education, and age achieved the default criteria ($F = .01$, tolerance $= .001$) and did not enter the equation. Shrinkage of the R^2 (.16) at the first step of the regression analysis was computed since the F of the b weight was significant only at this step. The estimated squared multiple correlation in the population was computed to be .13. The criterion variance accounted for by the surgery variable, using the test-retest coefficient as the lower-bound estimate of the reliability of the criterion, was computed to be .25. Hypothesis I was rejected.

Hypothesis II

Principal Component Analysis. The factor analysis with Varimax rotation resulted in three components. The first component, state board licensure examinations, was comprised of the following variables and their respective factor loadings: medicine, .91; pediatrics, .91; psychiatry, .77; surgery, .76; and obstetrics, .63. The variables which loaded highly on component II, biographical information, were age, .93; and work experience, .91. The variables of job satisfaction, .90, and leader behavior, .87, loaded highly on component III, attitude toward the work environment. The average interitem correlations ranged from .28 to .47 for the three components. The Spearman-Brown prophecy formula was used to estimate the alpha scale reliabilities for each component grouping. These were high enough to warrant retaining the three components.

Multiple Regression Analysis. The three components were used in a multiple regression analysis to determine the contribution of the largest components of nine selected variables to the variance of job performance. Education, a categorical variable, was omitted from the factor analysis (see Table 4).

TABLE 3
Stepwise Multiple Regression Analysis for the Raw Score Model[a]

Step Number	Independent Variable Entered	R	R^2	Increase in R^2	SE_{est}	df	F	Beta	b	SE_b	F_b
1	SBE-Surgery	.40	.16	.16	5.28	1,30	5.65[b]	−.73	−.56	.02	9.93[c]
2	Years of work experience	.49	.24	.08	5.09	2,29	4.61[b]	−.24	−.24	.02	1.62
3	SBE-Obstetrics	.57	.32	.08	4.89	3,28	4.49[c]	.32	.26	.02	2.42
4	SBE-Pediatrics	.61	.37	.05	4.79	4,27	4.05[b]	.46	.27	.02	2.17
5	LBDQ	.63	.40	.03	4.78	5,26	3.51[b]	−.22	−.10	.08	1.56
6	SBE-Medicine	.64	.41	.01	4.82	6,25	2.96[b]	−.23	−.14	.02	0.53
7	SBE-Psychiatry	.65	.42	.00	4.91	7,24	2.44[b]	−.04	.28	.02	0.03

[a] The dashed line after step 5 indicates increase of the standard error of estimate.
[b] $p < .05$.
[c] $p < .01$.

TABLE 4
Stepwise Multiple Regression Analysis Using a Data Reduction Model

Step Number	Component Entered	R	R^2	Increase in R^2	SE_{est}	df	F	Beta	b	SE_b	F_b
1	II. Biographical information	.28	.08	.08	5.52	1,30	2.60	−.28	−1.60	1.01	2.53
2	III. Attitude toward work environment	.32	.10	.02	5.54	2,29	1.68	−.16	−.88	1.01	.76
3	I. State board licensure examinations	.34	.12	.02	5.60	3,28	1.22	−.11	−.61	1.01	.36

Component II, biographical information, entered the regression equation on the first step. It explained 8 percent of the variance of job performance and had the highest b weight. Component III, attitude toward the work environment, entered the equation on the second step. There was a small increment in the R^2 and an increase in the standard error of estimate at this step. Component I, state board licensure examinations, entered the regression equation on the third step. Statistical significance for the F of the multiple correlation or the F of the b weight at each step was not achieved.

The second null hypothesis was supported. The nature of the criterion of job performance as measured by JPM scores seemed to favor the raw score model rather than a reduced-rank model. Perhaps as Elterich stated, "The relative usefulness of component, scale, or raw scores may depend upon the nature of the criterion."[28]

Limitations of the Study

Several factors limited the internal validity of this study. Multicollinearity limited the interpretation of the results of the multiple regression analyses used to investigate the study hypotheses. Several limitations can be attributed to the instruments used in this study. Initial validation studies of the JDI and the LBDQ did not include nurses in the samples. The range of scores on the JPM which was used to measure the dependent variable in this study was restricted; supervisors tended to rate highly job performance of their staff.

The systematic bias of supervisors in rating their staff nurses using the JPM was also investigated. The amount of scoring-error variance in the observed scores resulting from supervisory group membership of the sample was calculated. When Tukey's H.S.D. test was used for post hoc comparisons of mean differences on JPM ratings for the six supervisory groups, mean ratings for two supervisory groups were significantly different. With a larger sample, possibility of rater bias could have been examined more fully. Another persistent problem which limited the reliability of JPM scores was the work load of supervisory staff. Extensive time (one to two hours) was needed to rate a client's record using the JPM, and the pressure to complete the ratings may have increased scoring-error variance.

The generalizability of the findings of this study are limited because of the small size of the sample, use of volunteers rather than a random sample, and use of one agency as a source of volunteers. Also, no cross-validation sample was used to estimate the multiple correlation that would be obtained in the population of subjects.

Implications for Nursing

A Conceptual Framework for Evaluating Job Performance.
Using the ANA standards of quality care as the conceptual framework for the

development of the JPM provided the necessary conceptual structure to establish the content validity of the instrument. The broad scope of the standards permitted flexibility in defining related items that were appropriate for evaluating the job performance of nurses in a community health setting. Further consideration should be given to the use of the standards for developing quality assurance measures for nurses employed in any health care setting. While permitting creativity and diversity in defining items for various nursing roles, use of the standards would provide a unifying element for the profession by establishing the dimensions for the nursing process.

Correlates of Job Performance. Several variables appear to explain a portion of the variance of job performance for this sample of community health nurses: Intrinsic attributes such as work experience, cognitive knowledge of nursing content, and environmental factors such as the leadership behavior of superordinates. Influence of the selected independent variables in explaining job performance in this study was shown in the increase in the multiple correlation when these variables were included in the regression equation. The data supported the conclusion, reached by Haussmann et al. that the nursing profession should focus on a broad scope of variables, including environmental, organizational, and human relations dimensions, when investigating correlates of the quality of job performance of registered nurses.[29]

Judgmental Measurement of Job Performance. In this study, six supervisors acted as measuring instruments in judging staff on a record audit measure entitled the JPM. Wiggins discussed the issue of judgmental measurement of variables that are used in a regression equation: "Given the complex nature of the stimuli on which such judgments are based (i.e., human beings), it is difficult to obtain objective (nonjudgmental) criterion measures against which to validate the judgments."[30] In nursing, ratings of job performance using human, judgmental measurement is a necessary condition. The reliability issues of judgmental measurement were given serious consideration, but more questions were raised than answered. This study attempted to examine several components of error variance, in particular, the error variance that could be attributed to supervisory group membership. Additional studies of this nature should be undertaken in nursing to investigate the reliability of judges. Professional clinicians may not be more accurate in their judgments of others than lay persons.[31] Establishing the validity and the reliability of instruments to measure job performance of nurses is not enough. The larger issue of judgmental measurement by professionals or other persons is equally relevant.

Validity of Record Audit as a Quality Assurance Method. From the negative correlations found between the independent variables and the dependent variable of job performance, it may be tentatively concluded that other intervening variables influence the charting of care given by the professional nurse. Thus, record audits may not reflect the quality of care actually given by the nurse, but other factors such as time available for charting or perceived importance of charting by the nurse. Further research is needed to identify the intervening variables and suggest ways in which agencies can work to control them.

ABOUT THE AUTHOR

At the time of writing, Beverly Koerner, PhD, RN, was Associate Professor of Nursing und Education, and Chairman of the Nursing Department, University of Hartford, Hartford, Connecticut. The author acknowledges the assistance of the staff and administration of the Visiting Nurse Association of Hartford, Inc.

REFERENCES

1. E. D. Dyer, et al., "Can Job Performance Be Predicted from Biographical, Personality, and Administrative Climate Inventories?" *Nursing Research,* 21 (July-August 1972), 294–304; R. K. Haussmann, et al., *Monitoring Quality of Nursing Care: Part 2. Assessment and Study of Correlates,* DHEW Publ. No. (HRA) 76-7 (Washington, DC: U.S. Government Printing Office, 1976); and L. J. Welches et al., "Typological Prediction of Staff Nurse Performance Rating," *Nursing Research,* 23 (September-October 1974), 402–409.

2. Ludwig von Bertalanffy, *General Systems Theory* (New York: Braziller, 1969).

3. R. C. Jelinek, "A Structural Model for Patient Care Operation," *Health Services Research,* 2 (Fall 1967), 226–242.

4. Haussmann et al., *Monitoring Quality of Nursing Care: Part 2.*

5. E. D. Dyer, *Nurse Performance Description: Criteria, Predictors and Correlates* (Salt Lake City: University of Utah Press, 1967).

6. E. D. Dyer, et al., "What Are the Relationships of Quality Patient Care to Nurses' Performance, Biographical and Personality Variables?" *Psychological Reports,* 36 (February 1975), 255–266; Dyer et al., "Can Job Performance Be Predicted from Biographical, Personality, and Administrative Climate Inventories?" and Welches et al., "Typological Prediction of Staff Nurse Performance Rating."

7. Elizabeth Hagen and Luverne Wolff, *Nursing Leadership Behavior in General Hospitals* (New York: Teachers College, Columbia University, 1961); S. Hegyvary, "The Hospital Setting and Patient Care Outcomes: An Exploratory Study," unpublished doctoral dissertation, Vanderbilt University, Nashville, TN, 1974; and L. Kruse and R. Stogdill, *The Leadership Role of the Nurse* (Columbus: Ohio State University Research Foundation, 1973).

8. Haussmann et al., *Monitoring Quality of Nursing Care: Part 2.*

9. F. Herzberg, *Job Attitudes: Review of Research and Opinion* (Pittsburgh: Psychological Service of Pittsburgh, 1957); and J. W. Slocum, Jr., et al., "Analysis of Need Satisfaction and Job Performance among Professional and Paraprofessional Hospital Personnel," *Nursing Research,* 21 (July-August 1982), 338-342.

10. Haussmann et al., *Monitoring Quality of Nursing Care: Part 2.*

11. Welches et al., "Typological Prediction of Staff Nurse Performance Rating."

12. J. E. Gray, et al., "Do Graduates of Technical and Professional Nursing Programs Differ in Practice?" *Nursing Research,* 26 (September-October 1977), 368–373; and A. I. Meleis and K. M. Farrell, "Operation Concern: A Study of Senior Nursing Students in Three Nursing Programs," *Nursing Research,* 23 (November-December 1974), 461–468.

13. L. F. Nelson, "Competence of Nursing Graduates in Technical, Communicative, and Administrative Skills," *Nursing Research,* 27 (March-April 1978), 121–125.

14. Haussmann et al., *Monitoring Quality of Nursing Care: Part 2;* and Welches et al., "Typological Prediction of Staff Nurse Performance Rating."

15. Regina Dubs, "Comparison of Student Achievement with Performance Ratings of Graduates and State Board Examination Scores," *Nursing Research,* 24 (January-February 1975), 59–62, 64.

16. E. M. Brandt and B. H. Metheny, "Relationships between Measures of Student and Graduate Performance," *Nursing Research,* 17 (May-June 1968), 242–246.

17. Haussmann et al., *Monitoring Quality of Nursing Care: Part 2;* and M. W. Pryer and M. K. Distefano, Jr., "Perception of Leadership Behavior, Job Satisfaction, and Internal-External Locus of Control across Three Nursing Levels," *Nursing Research,* 20 (November-December 1971), 534–537.

18. Marlene Kramer, "Role Conceptions of Baccalaureate Nurses and Success in Hospital Nursing," *Nursing Research,* 19 (September-October 1970), 428–439.

19. American Nurses' Association, Congress for Nursing Practice, *A Plan for Implementation of the Standards of Nursing Practice* (Kansas City, MO: American Nurses' Association, 1975).

20. Doris Bloch, "Evaluation of Nursing Care in Terms of Process and Outcome: Issues in Research and Quality Assurance," *Nursing Research,* 24 (July-August 1975), 256–263.

21. P. C. Smith et al., *The Measurement of Satisfaction in Work and Retirement* (Chicago: Rand McNally & Co., 1969).

22. E. Fleishman, "A Leader Behavior Description for Industry," in R. Stogdill and A. Coons, eds., *Leader Behavior: Its Description and Measurement,* Monograph No. 88 (Columbus: Bureau of Business Research, Ohio State University, 1957), 103–119.

23. Haussmann et al., *Monitoring Quality of Nursing Care: Part 2.*

24. R. C. Jelinek et al., *A Methodology for Monitoring Quality of Nursing Care,* DHEW Publ. No. (HRA) 74–23 (Washington, DC: U.S. Government Printing Office, 1974).

25. A. L. Edwards, *Techniques of Attitude Scale Construction* (Englewood Cliffs, NJ: Prentice-Hall, 1979; originally published 1957).

26. R. Stogdill, *Manual for the Leader Behavior Description Questionnaire—Form XII* (Columbus: Bureau of Business Research, Ohio State University, 1963).

27. Smith et al., *The Measurement of Satisfaction in Work and Retirement.*

28. K. Elterich, "Three Regression Models: Their Relative Usefulness in Predicting College Achievement," unpublished doctoral dissertation, University of Connecticut, Storrs, 1976, p. 98.

29. Haussmann et al., *Monitoring Quality of Nursing Care: Part 2.*

30. J. S. Wiggins, *Personality and Prediction: Principles of Personality Assessment* Cambridge, MA: Addison-Wesley Publishing Co., 1973), p. 123.

31. Ibid.

Part 4

COMMUNITY-BASED DEMONSTRATIONS

Evaluation of Community-Oriented Long-Term Care Demonstration Projects

For many years the Department of Health and Human Services, and particularly the Health Care Financing Administration and the Administration on Aging, have supported research and demonstration to develop humane, efficient and effective long-term care services. It has been believed since the early 1970s that the frail aged often prefer community-oriented long-term care services to institutional care, and that with adequate supply and coordination of these services, potential exists for reducing the rate of growth in public expenditures for long-term care.[1] While demand by the aged and their families for a wider range of options in long-term care continues to grow,[2] and the supply of these services has shown a remarkable increase in many parts of the country,[3] controversy still exists concerning which approaches to the delivery and financing of community-oriented long-term care are most clinically and economically appropriate.

Excerpted from the introduction to *Evaluation of Community-Oriented Long-Term Care Demonstration Projects,* Health Care Financing Extramural Report, prepared by Berkeley Planning Associates, HCFA Pub. No. 0342 (Washington, DC: U. S. Government Printing Office, May 1987).
This project was funded at least in part with federal funds from the Department of Health and Human Services under Contract No. 500-80-0073. The contents do not necessarily reflect the views or policies of the Department of Health and Human Services, nor does mention of trade names, commercial products, or organizations imply endorsement by the U.S. government.

To explore different approaches to providing and financing publicly supported community-based long-term care, the Health Care Financing Administration (HCFA) in late 1980 sponsored a national evaluation of 13 projects demonstrating the provision of coordinated, community-oriented services to impaired and aged Medicare and Medicaid beneficiaries. These projects provided long-term care under Section 222 Medicare and/or Section 1115 Medicaid waivers that allow reimbursement for clients and for services not typically covered by Medicare and Medicaid. The projects tested whether various methods of case-managed, coordinated delivery of community-oriented health and social services could result in more cost-effective use of both institutional and non-institutional long-term care. The 13 projects included in the national evaluation were:

- The New York City Home Care Project (HCP);
- The Community Long-Term Care Project (LTCP) of North San Diego County;
- The ACCESS II program of Monroe County, New York;
- The South Carolina Community Long-Term Care Program (CLTCP);
- On Lok's Community Care Organization for Dependent Adults (CCODA), San Francisco;
- Project OPEN of Mount Zion Hospital, San Francisco;
- Triage II, Connecticut;
- Georgia's Alternative Health Services project (AHS);
- Wisconsin's Community Care Organization, Milwaukee;
- Florida's Pentastar project;
- California's Multipurpose Senior Services Project (MSSP);
- Oregon FIG/Waiver Continuum of Care Project for the Elderly; and
- The Texas ICF-II project.

This report summarizes major findings from the national evaluation, which was conducted by Berkeley Planning Associates (BPA) of Berkeley, California, with the assistance of two subcontractors: the Western Center for Health Planning in San Francisco and the Rehabilitation Research and Training Center in Aging, University of Pennsylvania.

GOALS AND SCOPE OF THE NATIONAL EVALUATION

The primary objectives of the national evaluation were:

1. To determine the clinical efficacy and cost-effectiveness of the demonstration projects in providing comprehensive care to chronically ill aged and other dependent adults;

2. To determine the impact of community-based long-term care services on the demonstration projects' selected clients, providers of both formal and informal care, local communities, and the federal government as the public ensurer of long-term care; and

3. To identify the key factors among the projects, relative to their host communities, that contribute to or impede the clinical efficacy and cost-effectiveness of the HCFA demonstrations.

As part of the overall national evaluation, seven major levels of analysis were undertaken: (1) analysis of key project characteristics and classification of intervention approaches; (2) analysis of targeting goals and client group composition; (3) analysis of participant outcomes (functional status and mortality); (4) analysis of service utilization and costs; (5) analysis of case management functions and costs; (6) analysis of informal supports; and (7) analysis of diffusion of innovations from the demonstrations. Table 1 lists the demonstration projects which were included in each level of analysis.

During its three years, the national evaluation has undergone considerable narrowing of its focus in response to resource constraints and further refinement of policy concerns in long-term care. At the request of HCFA and the demonstration projects, analysis of participant outcomes and cost-effectiveness received priority throughout the study. In order to conduct an in-depth evaluation in these two priority areas, the original scope of this component of the evaluation was narrowed from 13 projects to focus on three primary and three secondary projects.

The three primary evaluation sites identified by HCFA early in the study were: the New York City Home Care Project (HCP), the Long-Term Care Project (LTCP) of North San Diego County, and the ACCESS II program of Monroe County, New York. Thse projects were chosen for primary evaluations because they lacked independent research components or had inadequate resources available for an evaluation. Since the ACCESS II project did not become operational until November 1982 and is anticipated to continue serving clients until July 1986, even preliminary analyses of the program (based on a quasi-experimental design including comparative samples in two other upstate New York counties) will not be available until late 1984.

Three other projects were selected for inclusion in the in-depth analysis of participant outcomes and cost-effectiveness: the South Carolina Community Long-Term Care Program (CLTCP); On Lok's Community Care Organization for Dependent Adults (CCODA), San Francisco; and Project OPEN of Mt. Zion Hospital, San Francisco. These three programs were selected because they represent important contrasts to the primary projects with respect to their intervention designs, target populations and host communities.

While not included in the detailed analyses of participant and cost impacts, the remaining demonstration projects were used in specifying models of alternative long-term care intervention, target group definitions, or case management systems. Three of these programs, Triage, Georgia's Alternative Health Services Project

TABLE 1
Projects Included in the Various Levels of Analysis Undertaken for the National Evaluation

Analysis of Key Project Characteristics and Classification of Intervention Approaches	Analysis of Targeting Goals and Client Group Composition	Analysis of Participant Outcomes: Functional Status and Mortality	Analysis of Service Utilization and Costs	Analysis of Case Management Function Costs	Analysis of Informal Supports	Analysis of Diffusion of Innovations from the Demonstrations
New York City HCP	New York City HCP	New York City HCP	New York City HCP	New York City HCP	New York City HCP	South Carolina CLTCP
San Diego LTCP	San Diego LTCP	San Diego LTCP	San Diego LTCP	San Diego LTCP	San Diego LTCP	MSSP
South Carolina CLTCP	South Carolina CLTCP	South Carolina CLTCP	South Carolina CLTCP	South Carolina CLTCP	South Carolina CLTCP	ACCESS
On Lok CCODA	On Lok CCODA	On Lok CCODA	On Lok CCODA	On Lok CCODA		
Project OPEN	Project OPEN	Project OPEN	Project OPEN	Project OPEN		
ACCESS II	ACCESS II	ACCESS II[a]	ACCESS II[a]			
Triage II	Triage					
Wisconsin CCO	Wisconsin CCO					
Florida Pentastar	Florida Pentastar					
MSSP	MSSP					
Georgia AHS						
Oregon FIG/Waiver						
Texas ICF-II						

[a]ACCESS II findings on participant outcomes and service utilization and costs will be availalable as a separate report in 1986.

(AHS), and the Wisconsin Community Care Organization (CCO), were excluded from the in-depth evaluation because adequate primary and secondary analyses of their experiences have been reported elsewhere.[4] The results of these oldest programs are well known and are referenced where appropriate. The State of Florida's Pentastar project and the State of California's Multipurpose Senior Services Project (MSSP) were excluded from the in-depth evaluation because comprehensive state-sponsored evaluations are underway. The Oregon FIG/Waiver and the Texas ICF-II projects were excluded because of the lack of comparable experimental or quasi-experimental research designs. However, BPA has received a large data base compiled by the State of Texas concerning the demonstration, and hopes to analyze that data if federal support is forthcoming.

The narrowing of the participant outcome and cost-effectiveness evaluation from 13 to five projects (which excludes ACCESS II data that is not available at this time, but will be incorporated at a later date when available) affords the opportunity for greater detail and specificity in the study of those demonstrations included. This focus does, of course, limit the generalizability of study findings. On the other hand, components of the overall evaluation which included projects not featured in the detailed analyses of participant and cost outcomes provided a unique opportunity to document and study the variations in coordinated community-oriented long-term care programs.

One of the most serious problems facing policymakers in developing national long-term care policy (especially concerning community-oriented care) is the dearth of solid information on how long-term care services are delivered. BPA's description of each of the HCFA demonstration projects, documentation of case management practices, and analysis of demonstration features are important contributions to the effort to fill this gap in knowledge and form the basis for interpretation of the quantitative study findings.

In this way, material from a number of community care approaches has strengthened the interpretation of data from the five projects that were selected for the in-depth evaluation of participant and cost outcomes. This interpretative background, as well as the analytic approach firmly based on individual program evaluation, distinguishes this evaluation from prior research in long-term care reform.

THE ANALYTIC APPROACH

An approach—sometimes advocated, but rejected for use in this study—to analyzing data across a number of research projects is to pool the data from various demonstrations into a single analysis. This approach can be inappropriate for a number of reasons, the two foremost of these being: (a) the projects may be very different from one another on key variables such as client characteristics, range of services, and cost of care; and (b) participants at different sites may be drawn from different populations (e.g., Medicare and/or Medicaid) and may not be comparable on relevant dimensions such as income, living arrangements, and level of disability.

In this study of long-term care programs, there were a number of factors which precluded the pooling of data from the various demonstration projects into a single analysis. For example, there were variations in individual project goals, intervention methods, community contexts and service package configurations, as well as differences in the research designs, assessment variables and procedures, and data acquisition methods.

Because of these variations in individual projects, a two-stage analytical approach was used for the cross-site analysis. During the first stage, the best-available approach to analysis of individual data for each project was pursued. All appropriate measures within the relevant domains (e.g., functional status, participant well-being, unmet needs, and service costs) were utilized, and quantitative analysis of program impact based on treatment and comparative group differences was undertaken. Qualitative data on program design and intervention approaches were used to guide the interpretation of the findings.

In the second stage of the analysis, which focused on participant outcomes and cost-effectiveness across five selected projects, only those data measures that were available across projects were utilized.[5] However, the best available approach to analysis of each individual project's data was still used. The goal was to find the best estimates of program impact for individual projects, focusing on types of impact measures (e.g., functional status and cost variables) of concern to policymakers and program designers. Variations in the direction and magnitude of effects across projects were then described and compared using both quantitative and qualitative data, as appropriate. In some of the cross-cutting analyses, a descriptive approach was used to compare demonstration projects. Large differences between the projects as well as trends and patterns are discussed, but statistical tests of significance were not performed across projects, due to the limitations in the standardization of variables across sites.

The overall analysis plan has been guided by the general concern in the long-term care field and in HCA that advocacy for community-based long-term care has too often been based largely on qualitative data and nonrigorous research. Consequently, throughout the report, the primary analyses focused on quantitative data and employed a number of rigorous research techniques. First, data from each project's comparison group has been used consistently to assess whether community-based alternatives to traditional long-term care have reduced costs and achieved better participant outcomes. Second, within each project's data set, baseline differences in participants' functional status and other characteristics have been controlled to ensure that seemingly apparent program impacts are not due to differences between the treatment and comparative groups served. Thus, the analyses have excluded, to the maximum extent possible, effects that are due to the type of participants served rather than to the nature of the care. Third, the differences found have been subjected to statistical significance testing to ensure that the findings reported and emphasized for their substantive importance are not simply findings that might arise due to chance. Fourth, strict, academic standards have been used in judging statistical significance, i.e., .05 significance levels, which make only very strong findings emerge as "significant." Finally, throughout the report, statistically significant findings are emphasized, and the discussion of overall trends and patterns which are not statistically significant is clearly identified as such.

SUMMARY OF MAJOR PERFORMANCE EVALUATION FINDINGS

The five demonstration projects selected for an in-depth analysis of participant outcomes and cost-effectiveness, with the size of their treatment and comparative group samples are:

	Sample	
Project	Treatment Group	Comparative Group
New York City HCP	504	200
On Lok CCODA	69	70
Project OPEN	220	118
San Diego LTCP	555	328
South Carolina CLTCP	539	553

These five projects vary along key program characteristics, which can be expected to have an impact on participant and cost outcomes. The key program dimensions are the intervention approach, the targeting goal, and the clients' level of functional impairment.

The five sample projects represent three different intervention approaches: direct control of institutional admissions (South Carolina CLTCP); consolidation of service delivery in a single agency (On Lok CCODA); and upgrading the home care package (San Diego LTCP, New York City HCP, and Project OPEN).

With respect to targeting goals and client characteristics, the five projects represent two different types of targeting goals, while the client population includes individuals at three different levels of functional impairment. The South Carolina CLTCP and On Lok CCODA both targeted clients from a variety of long-term care settings (i.e., hospital, nursing home, or home) with need for either institutional or community services. These two projects also served clients who were severely impaired relative to the other demonstration projects. The New York City HCP, San Diego LTCP, and Project OPEN all targeted their services to clients in the community who needed community services.

However, the level of functional impairment found among clients in these three projects varied considerably. The New York City HCP served a severely impaired client population, while the San Diego LTCP served a moderately impaired client population, and Project OPEN served a client population with minor impairment relative to the other demonstration projects. These five projects are fairly representative of the range of characteristics found among the 13 demonstration projects included in the overall evaluation.

Based on data from the five projects selected for the in-depth evaluation, the principal findings are summarized below.

- In general, the results of the demonstration's impact on participants' functional status were mixed. Change in functional status over time was assessed in three areas: Activities of Daily Living (ADL), Instrumental Activities of Daily Living (IADL), and mental status (MSQ). Statistically significant program impacts related to change in functional status were only found in four projects.

    —In the On Lok program, after controlling for baseline differences, a significant program effect was found on the IADL measure at the 12-month reassessment. Relative to the comparison group, the treatment group improved in IADL.

    —In Project OPEN, controlling for the level of functioning at baseline, a significant treatment effect was noted on the MSQ measure at the six-month reassessment.

    —In the San Diego and New York City projects, after controlling for baseline differences, a significant treatment effect was found on the mental status measure at the 12-month reassessment.

- Although there were few statistically significant program impacts related to participants' functional status, there was an overall pattern for the treatment groups to have more favorable participant outcomes than the comparative groups. In addition, an assessment of change in the functional status of individual clients over time indicated that each of the five projects was successful in maintaining or improving the functional status of more than one-half of their client population.

- While there were no statistically significant program impacts related to mortality, in the majority of the projects, a smaller proportion of the treatment group than the comparative group died within the 12-month study period.

Overall, the findings indicate that community-oriented long-term care provides services that are no less effective than the services provided by the existing institutionally oriented long-term care system. To the extent that community-oriented long-term care is preferred by the elderly, their families, and society at large for reasons related to societal values, then community-oriented care is not less effective than the traditional long-term care system.

In terms of the evaluation's cost-effectiveness studies, analysis was carried out in the five projects to permit development of a standard unit of measurement for program impacts. the anlaysis expresses the marginal costs of the demonstration in terms of the additional hospital or nursing home days that would need to be used (or saved) by the treatment or comparative samples in order to equalize their total public costs during the first year after project enrollment. The principal findings are summarized below.

- From the perspective of project intervention designs, results suggest that both the direct diversion of nursing home applicants through pre-admission screening and expanded community services represented by the South Carolina CLTCP, and the consolidated model of long-term care represented by On Lok, are associated with reductions in traditional Medicaid or Medicare service use that are not completely offset by the incremental costs of the demonstration (e.g., case management and waivered services). In short, these two projects "broke even" in terms of public costs and showed some likelihood of constraining growth in public payments.

- In contrast, the San Diego LTCP and New York City's HCP, both representing an intervention designed to upgrade the home care package, did not break even. In both cases, the high costs of the waivered service packages (including case management) were not associated with reduced acute care and nursing home use, or reduction in overall costs. On the other hand, Project OPEN, with a similar intervention design to San Diego's LTCP and the New York City HCP, showed some likelihood of breaking even. The project, a hospital-based consortium of providers, was able to introduce some control of Medicare-reimbursed hospitalizations, without excessively increasing public costs through the waivered services. It should be noted, however, that Project OPEN's comparative group used nearly the same amount of the expanded community services as did the treatment group. The comparative group members either purchased these services out-of-pocket or received them through other public sources, without the assistance of case management. In a different, less service-rich community environment than San Francisco, such services might not be available to the normal population represented by a control group; thus, the differential impact between a treatment and a comparative group might well be larger.

In many respects the findings from this national evaluation confirm findings of several recent studies concerning the cost-effectiveness of community-oriented long-term care.

- There is some support for the contention that coordinated community-oriented long-term care programs can reduce nursing home use, *if* projects target individuals as they apply for nursing home admission or are at the SNF certifiable level of care.

- The demonstration projects, in most cases, did not impact acute care use. In a few cases acute hospitalization increased under the demonstration.

- For most of the demonstrations, the expanded service systems are more expensive to the public in the short run than the existing system of care, given the lack of targeting to those most at-risk of institutionalization. However, within a break-even context, hopeful findings for cost containment and reduction emerged for two projects, the South Carolina CLTCP and On Lok, which, in fact, served individuals with demonstrated risk of nursing home placement.

Finally, several of the findings from this study point to important factors related to cost-effectiveness that have not been emphasized in previous studies of community-oriented long-term care.

- Project variations in the likelihood of nursing home use (and, in fact, use of all medical services) cannot be attributed to variations in functioning, as measured by familiar scales such as Activities of Daily Living or mental status. To the contrary, with the exception of the prediction of nursing home use in the South Carolina CLTCP and home health care use in the San Diego LTCP, case mix factors explained less than 5 percent of the variance in any measure of service use or reimbursement. This finding is partially an artifact of the low levels of nursing home use in most projects, but still indicates that other factors, such as an individual's relationship to the system of care (e.g., community or institutional residence at baseline), can be major determinants of service utilization and costs.

- Although the New York City Home Care Project identified one of the most highly impaired samples, the clients made little use of nursing homes. The New York City HCP findings (like San Diego LTCP's findings) suggest that locating frail elders who hve service needs (in fact, in some cases, severe service needs) in the community does not automatically result in clear patterns of reduced use of institutional long-term care and associated cost savings. Individuals such as those served by the New York City and San Diego projects are not at risk of institutionalization only because of service needs.

- Informal caregivers (i.e., family and friends) offer a major source of assistance for the impaired elderly and, as such, represent the foundation upon which cost-effective community long-term care interventions should be based. Findings from this study indicate erosion of the informal support systems was, to some extent, evident in each of the demonstration projects studied. In the South Carolina project, however, where the informal caregivers were directly included in service planning and where the service plans for individuals explicitly were designed to augment the informal support systems, there was not a reduction in the level of effort by the informal caregivers, but merely a shift in the kinds of activities undertaken. In the San Diego and New York City projects, where there was not the explicit attention given to the informal support systems, there were, in contrast, both declines in the overall types of care given by informal providers and in the overall levels of care and effort given.

- The findings from the informal support study also suggest informal care outcomes are closely related to the characteristics of a program's target population. In South Carolina, where expanded community long-term care benefits were offered to clients for whom nursing home placement was imminent, supplementation of the informal support system was the most successful.

REFERENCES

1. H. Kistin and R. Morris, "Alternatives to Institutional Care for the Elderly and Disabled," *Gerontologist,* 2(2) (1972); M. Kaufman, "Social Policy and Long-Term Care of the Aged," *Social Work* (March 1980); and B. Gurland, R. Bennett, and D. Wilder, "Reevaluating the Place of Evaluation in Planning for Alternatives to Institutional Care for the Elderly, *Journal of Social Issues,* 37(3) (1981), 51-89.

2. U. S. General Accounting Office, "The Elderly Should Benefit from Expanded Home Health Care but Increasing These Services Will Not Ensure Cost Reductions," report to the Chairman, Committee on Labor and Human Response, U. S. Senate, December 7, 1982.

3. For example, the availability of adult day health care programs grew by 300 percent between 1977 and 1979. U. S. Department of Health and Human Services, *Directory of ADHC Centers* (Washington, DC: Department of Health & Human Services, Health Care Financing Administration, September 1980).

4. The results of these demonstrations were reviewed in detail in Appendix D of Berkeley Planning Associates, "Preliminary Report on Work in Progress," *Evaluation of Coordinated Community-Oriented Long-Term Care Demonstration Projects* (Berkeley, CA: Berkeley Planning Associates, October 1982), and are available on request.

5. Development of the common data set is described in Chapters 4 through 6 and Appendices A and C of the full report.

Part 5

INSTRUMENT DEVELOPMENT

Health-Specific Family Coping Index
for Noninstitutional Care

Thomas Choi, LaVohn Josten, and Mary Lou Christensen

INTRODUCTION

An instrument that assesses how well a patient's family is coping or functioning will influence the decision of whether that patient stays at home or is institutionalized. In turn, this decision will affect the cost and efficiency of the health care delivery system.

After reviewing 19 indices designed to gauge patient functioning, a task force of public health nurses selected three indices as the most appropriate for use by public health personnel on the basis of their practicality and methodological rigor or potential for such rigor. The Richmond/Hopkins Family Coping Index[1] was one of three selected, and further tests on the index were conducted to ensure its reliability in assessing family coping.[2]

The usefulness of the Family Coping Index has been amply covered.[3] This paper illustrates how the accuracy and consistency of the Family Coping Index can be further improved.

Reprinted with permission from *American Journal of Public Health,* 73 (November 1983), pp. 1275-1277, copyright © 1983, American Journal of Public Health.

This project was supported in part by BRSG 2S07 RR 05448-18 awarded by the Biomedical Research Support Grant Program, Division of Research Resources, National Institutes of Health. An earlier version of this paper was presented at the 110th Annual Meeting of the American Public Health Association, Montreal, Canada, November 1982.

METHODS

Experienced public health personnel (raters) were given an explicit set of instructions (operations manual) on the use of the Family Coping Index. They
were then randomly assigned to groups, each of which rated the level of coping
in a common set of patients and their families using two coping instruments.
Within and between group ratings were then tested for consistency and the instruments were tested for consistency in measuring coping. Results from this
process were compared with results from the earlier study that did not use the
operations manual.[4]

The construction of an operations manual (see Fig. 1) was intended to clarify
the original instructions provided by Freeman and Lowe,[5] which were aimed
at rating family coping in nine domains: (1) physical independence; (2)
therapeutic competence; (3) knowledge of health condition; (4) application of
principles of general hygiene; (5) health care attitude; (6) emotional competence;
(7) family living patterns; (8) physical environment; and (9) use of community
resources.

Clarifications included differentiating the nine domains—the boundaries of
which were previously amorphous—and clearly defining each level of coping
so that appropriate ratings could be assigned. The manual's specific modifications to the original instructions were: (1) adjusting the nine subscales (one for
each domain) from a range of 0-4 to 1-5[6] (this linear transformation was
psychologically important to public health personnel using the subscales because
"0" represented nothing and "1" represented a meaningful degree on a
continuum); (2) adding definitions of coping across and within domains for
all five levels instead of just for levels 1, 3 and 5 as in the original instructions;
(3) distinguishing types of coping into disease/disability and health promotion
categories; and (4) clarifying what does not belong in each domain.

To help assess measurement accuracy, a second instrument called "The
General Aptitude Family Coping Index" (with brief instructions) was constructed
(with the help of an expert panel) to gauge the family's potential for coping
as stressful life events occur (see Fig. 2). Like the Health-Specific Family Coping
Index (HSFCI), the Aptitude Index is made up of nine questions with five intervals each. The nine constructs that make up the General Aptitude Family
Coping Index are a family's (1) recognition of need for help; (2) clarity of perceptions; (3) supportive exchange; (4) stress level; (5) pattern of coping; (6) fulfillment of roles; (7) energy level; (8) reality orientation; and (9) participative decision making.

Both instruments ask the rater to assess how a family is coping in the nine
specific health domains, and how ready that family is to cope generally.

Seven vignettes of family coping based on real patient cases were used as test
cases. These vignettes were selected from existing cases to simulate intervals along
the full range of family coping levels—from coping very well to coping very
poorly—in each of the nine domains. Using a modified Delphi approach, these

FIGURE 1
Operations Manual for the Health-Specific Family Coping Index

The Health-Specific Family Coping Index consists of nine domains: physical independence, therapeutic competence, knowledge of health condition, application of principles of general hygiene, health care attitude, emotional competence, family living patterns, physical environment, and use of community resources. Definitions of scaling cues for five levels of coping are described for use across all nine domains. For each of the nine domains, the operations manual includes definitions of what type of functioning is included in this domain, clarification as to what does and does not constitute coping in each domain, a description of each of the five levels of coping, and an example of disease/disability and health promotion for each of the five levels. Scoring each patient for each of the nine domains is recorded on a scoring sheet in the patient record. *

The following is an example of instructions given for one domain of coping in the comprehensive operations manual:

COPING DOMAIN: KNOWLEDGE OF HEALTH CONDITION

Definition

This parameter measures the family's knowledge of the facts. It is concerned with the particular health condition or developmental change that is the occasion for care. This category documents the patient's and his/her family's knowledge of that condition including the principles underlying the recommendation.

Clarification

This category does not include how family members apply that knowledge (therapeutic competence) or how they apply knowledge of general hygiene, nor does it include their attitude toward that knowledge.

Scale

1. The family is totally uninformed or misinformed about the condition.

   Examples
   a. *Disease/Disability*—Family mistakenly believes that heart disease is cured when patient no longer has chest pain.
   b. *Health Promotion*—A pregnant woman does not know any of the hazards to her fetus.

2. The family has vague knowledge of principles of condition.

   Examples
   a. *Disease/Disability*—Family misunderstands heart disease to be caused by something the patient eats.
   b. *Health Promotion*—A pregnant woman knows she needs a good diet during pregnancy, but does not know any specific requirements.

3. The family has some general knowledge of the disease or condition, but only partially understands the specifics.

---

*For copies of the Health-Specific Family Coping Index and the accompanying operations manual, contact: Mary Lou Christensen, Associate Director, Ramsey County Public Health Nursing Service, 910 American Center Building, 150 East Kellogg Boulevard, St. Paul, MN 55101.

FIG. 1 (continued)

Examples
   a. *Disease/Disability*—Family of heart patient knows of the changes in the patient's life-style necessitated by the condition, but is not aware that the support of family members will be necessary the rest of his/her life.
   b. *Health Promotion*—Pregnant woman understands some body changes, but does not know most of the danger signs.

4. The family knows the majority of basic components of health/illness, some of the signs of complications, and when to seek medical care.

Examples
   a. *Disease/Disability*—Family of heart patient knows the life-style changes are permanent, but does not understand rationale underlying symptoms to be reported.
   b. *Health Promotion*—Family of pregnant woman understands physiological changes and most danger signs.

5. Family knows salient facts about disease/developmental stage, complications, and when to seek appropriate medical care.

Examples
   a. *Disease/Disability*—Family of heart patient knows life-style changes are permanent, and they understand the rationale underlying the symptoms to be reported.
   b. *Health Promotion*—Family of pregnant woman understands physiological changes and danger signs.

FIGURE 2
The General Aptitude Family Coping Index

The General Aptitude Family Coping Index consists of nine questions that assess a family's aptitude for successfully coping with life events. A five-level scale is used to score aptitude as reflected by each of the nine questions (1 = never; 2 = occasionally; 3 = sometimes; 4 = frequently; 5 = always). These nine questions are:

1. Do they recognize the need for and accept help?
2. Do they accurately preceive their life situation including their health condition, and the current and potential results of the actions of themselves and others?
3. Do they have reciprocal support relationships?
4. Is their stress level low?
5. Did they use constructive methods in coping with previous life changes and stressful situations?
6. Do they fulfill family and societal roles?
7. Is the physical condition, including energy level, of each family member good?
8. Do they balance the need to be confident in their own and their family members' abilities with a realistic acceptance of their own and their family members' limitations?
9. Do they have mutuality in communication, interaction, and decision making within the family?

vignettes or case descriptions were confirmed by an expert panel as realistic and representative of patient situations. Real life ambiguities were retained in the vignettes so that no vignette portrayed a setting where the coping was clearly at a uniform level for all domains.

Fifty public health/home baccalaureate-trained nurses equally distributed in two different agencies agreed to participate in rating the seven vignettes. Raters ranged in age from 25 to 60, with a median age of 30. Years of health care experience ranged from 2 to 38 years, with 6.3 the median. Years of experience in home care ranged from 1 to 33 years, with a median of 3.2 years. Years with the present agency ranged from 1 to 19 years, with 2.7 the median.

Each rater was randomly assigned to one of the three groups. Raters in Group 1 individually and independently rated the vignettes using only HSFCI; raters in Group 2 rated the vignettes using only the Aptitude Index, and raters in Group 3 rated the vignettes using both indices.

RESULTS

As Table 1 illustrates, regardless of how the raters were grouped, there was high consistency within and between groups in using the indices to rate family coping.

The level of agreement for each vignette (judged by the relative size of variances) varied according to the level of coping portrayed. Extremes of coping (high and low levels) tended to bring about the most agreement.

Table 2 shows that the HSFCI replicated the one-factor solution that Choi and Strohschein had found earlier.[7] But the HSFCI explained markedly more variance (83 percent) than the original Family Coping Index (59 percent).

TABLE 1
Interrater Reliability[a] by Agency, Group, and Instrument

	Health-Specific Family Coping Index	General Aptitude Family Coping Index
Both agencies—all groups	.99	.99
Agency A		
Group 1	.98	NA
Group 2	NA	.99
Group 3	.97	.97
Agency B		
Group 1	.98	NA
Group 2	NA	.97
Group 3	.98	.98

[a]Cronbach's alpha.

TABLE 2
Health-Specific Family Coping Index Factor Analysis — One Factor Solution[a]

Dimension	Factor Loading
1 Physical independence	.91
2 Therapeutic competence	.90
3 Knowledge of health condition	.71
4 Hygiene application	.94
5 Health attitude	.91
6 Emotional competence	.96
7 Family living patterns	.94
8 Physical environment	.90
9 Use of resources	.92

[a]Varimax rotated one factor matrix for the Family Coping Index. Percent of variance explained = 83%.

The correlation between the HSFCI and the Aptitude Index (.94) was also highly significant.

A summary score of the HSFCI for each patient or client can be easily obtained by summing the subscores in each of the nine domains, with 9 and 45 being the minimum and the maximum total score. This summing procedure weighs each domain uniformly because of the homogeneous factor loadings in all but one of the nine areas (see Table 2).

DISCUSSION

The high interrater reliability shown in Table 1 indicates that the instructions and operationalization of the instruments are effective in eliminating ambiguity. The replication of the single factor solution indicates that the Family Coping Index is quite stable across time, place, and raters.

The 83 percent explained variance of the HSFCI with the aid of the operations manual, as compared to 59 percent without a manual, suggests that the operations manual adds to the efficiency and accuracy in measuring the underlying construct of health-specific family coping. This interpretation has to be tempered by the presence of competing explanations, however. The earlier study rated case situations face-to-face while this study rated case vignettes. On the other hand, the diversity of raters in this study (raters were from two different agencies rather than just one), would be expected to attenuate the high percent of variance explained by the HSFCI.

Some uncertainties remain concerning the application of the instrument from rating case vignettes to rating face-to-face case situations. We believe that this is not likely to be a problem considering the comparability in results between this study and the face-to-face study conducted earlier.

Another concern we addressed was that of congruence between two different instruments both purportedly measuring coping. The high correlation between the two instruments gives us confidence that the common domain of coping was probably measured by the indices.

Although coping levels can be measured by a summary score, it is not clear whether the HSFCI should be weight-adjusted for differences in age, sex, race, and family type. Further, the consistency in factor loadings across the items suggests that the index can be made more parsimonious by deleting some of the items. To determine which items to delete and which to retain is easy to do mathematically but far more complicated if a consensus is to be reached among public health care delivery personnel. These issues remain to be addressed by future research.

ABOUT THE AUTHORS

At the time of writing, Thomas Choi, PhD, was at the Center for Health Services Research, University of Minnesota, Minneapolis. LaVohn Josten, MN, RN, FAAN, was at InterStudy, University of Minnesota. Mary Lou Christensen, MPH, RN, was Associate Director, Ramsey County Public Health Nursing Service, St. Paul, Minnesota.

REFERENCES

1. R. B. Freeman and M. Lowe, "A Method for Appraising Family Public Health Nursing Need," *American Journal of Public Health,* 53 (1963), 47-52; R. B. Freeman and M. Lowe, *Richmond/Hopkins Family Coping Index* (Richmond: Richmond, Virginia, Instructive Visiting Nurse Association, and Baltimore, MD: John Hopkins University School of Hygiene and Public Health, 1964) (mimeographed); and R. B. Freeman and W. B. Heinrich, *Community Health Nursing Practice* (2nd ed.; Philadelphia: W. B. Saunders, 1981).

2. T. Choi and S. Strohschein, "Health Status Measures for Public Health Nursing Use," unpublished manuscript (Minneapolis: University of Minnesota, Center for Health Services Research, 1982).

3. Freeman and Heinrich, *Community Health Nursing Practice.*

4. Choi and Strohschein, "Health Status Measures for Public Health Nursing Use."

5. Freeman and Lowe, *Richmond/Hopkins Family Coping Index.*

6. This change was independently made by Freeman and Heinrich in *Community Health Nurse Practice,* after the Family Coping Index was first reported by Freeman and Lowe in *Richmond/Hopkins Family Coping Index,* in 1964.

7. Choi and Strohschein, "Health Status Measures for Public Health Nursing Use."

Quality of Life as a Cancer Nursing Outcome Variable

Geraldine V. Padilla and Marcia M. Grant

Quality of life is an appropriate outcome for evaluating the impact of cancer nursing care. The phrase "quality of life" refers to that which makes life worth living and connotes the caring aspects of nursing, because nursing is concerned not only with survival and decreased morbidity, but with the whole patient. In caring for cancer patients, the nurse's role is frequently one of helping the patient to manage the side effects of therapy and to adjust to the permanent changes in body image, function, and appearance. The quality of the patient's survival may be associated not only with the inherent personal strength of the patient, but also with how well the nurse is able to help the patient with needed changes and adjustments.

As a research construct used as a dependent variable measure of the impact of nursing process, quality of life presents interesting theoretical and measurement challenges. These challenges are intrinsically linked once the operational definition used to measure quality of life is based on theoretical notions of the construct and how it is an effect of the nursing process. The problems faced

Reprinted with permission of Aspen Publishers, Inc., from *Advances in Nursing Science,* 8 (October 1985), pp. 45-58, copyright © 1985, Aspen Systems Corporation.

The studies on which this article is based were supported in part by grant NU00849 from the Division of Nursing, Bureau of Health Professions of the Health Resources and Services Administration, Rockville, Maryland.

by investigators using quality of life as an outcome variable include: theoretical insufficiency, definitional ambiguity, measurement insensitivity, and lack of population norms and fluctuations for targeted ill populations such as cancer patients.[1] It is the purpose of this article to present a multidimensional definition of quality of life, to present evidence that defines the reliability and validity of the approach, and to test a possible conceptual model for applying this approach to other cancer nursing research questions.

QUALITY OF LIFE DEFINITION

Nursing has provided the following operational definitions of quality of life. Laborde and Powers rated quality of life on the Cantril self-anchoring scale in relation to past, present, and future life satisfaction.[2] Young and Longman defined quality of life as the degree of satisfaction with perceived present life circumstances as measured on a 6-point scale.[3] Lewis chose to define quality of life as the degree to which one has self-esteem, a purpose in life, and minimal anxiety as measured by three separate instruments yielding three distinct socres.[4] Burckhardt defined quality of life as a composite score of the degree to which one perceives that life's quality is good, that life is satisfying, that the individual has physical and material well-being, good relations with others, and the ability to participate in social/community/civic activities, and that the individual has personal development, fulfillment, and recreation.[5]

The Karnofsky scale is the most common quality of life measure for cancer patients participating in clinical trials.[6] This scale measures the patient's ability to participate in physical activity; it is composed of 100 points, with 100 representing the highest activity level, and 0 representing death. The Karnofsky scale form is filled out by the physician. The scale was designed specifically to measure functional performance, especially for patients undergoing cancer chemotherapy research.[7] The advantages of this scale are that it is familiar to many clinicians and it has been used by many investigators so that normative data are available and comparisons across studies are possible. Its disadvantages are that it measures only one dimension of quality of life (i.e., physical functioning), and that it is scored by the physician and does not reflect the patient's perceived quality of life.

Thus nurses have viewed quality of life as both a unidimensional and multidimensional construct whereas the most common cancer patient quality of life measure is unidimensional. Both views may be correct. Certainly it is possible to ask a person to evaluate his or her quality of life on the basis of one question and the score is both valid and reliable.[8] However, a person's evaluation of the degree to which life is worth living is based on a number of criteria, and therefore, the multidimensional definition of quality of life is also correct and may be a more appropriate cancer nursing outcome measure. The studies reported here focus on the development of an instrument called the Quality of Life Index (QLI). The tool provides a multidimensional operational definition of quality of life and is expected to be sensitive to the nursing process being evaluated.

STUDY 1

Items selected for the first QLI study were based on a definition of quality of life that included the dimensions of performance (i.e., physical functioning), personal attitudes or affective states, well-being, and support. It was felt that because these aspects of quality of life are subjective, they are rated best by the individual patient. Thus a linear analogue scale of 100 millimeters was used as the response modality for each item because it provides a continuous measure of a subjective state. A word denoting extremes in response anchors each end of the scale. The patient marks an "X" on the line at the place that represents how he or she feels about the specific item. The mark is then transposed to a number from 1 to 100 using a millimeter ruler, with 1 denoting the poorest quality of life and 100 the best quality of life.

Items for the first QLI included several questions tested in a pilot study by Presant et al.,[9] as well as others, reflecting performance, personal attitudes or affective state, well-being, and support. A necessary limitation in developing the QLI was the focus on those aspects of quality of life that are relevant to the nursing care of cancer patients. Thus the approach used to select items for quality of life assessment did not include broad societal problems on which nursing care has little, if any, impact. A total of 14 items comprised the first QLI tool. Items anchored by the words "none" and "normal for me" included statements about strength, appetite, work, eating, sexual satisfaction, sleep, fun, satisfaction in life, and the feeling of being useful. The other five items were on pain, nausea, vomiting, general quality of life, and medical costs, and were anchored by extremes such as "none" to "excruciating" for pain.

Reliability and validity testing was done with four groups: cancer chemotherapy inpatients (48), cancer chemotherapy outpatients (43), cancer radiation therapy outpatients (39), and nonpatients (48). A complete report of Study 1 can be found in Padilla et al.[10]

Reliability of the first QLI was established via test-retest procedures. The patients were retested within 24 hours of the original testing, and the nonpatients were retested anywhere from 24 hours to 1 week later. A detailed description of this reliability testing is reported elsewhere and indicates that the instrument was reliable, especially for cancer patients.[11] The scores on retesting were significantly more stable for nonpatients and chemotherapy outpatients than for the other two groups. This was as expected, because the chemotherapy inpatients and the radiation outpatients were more vulnerable to daily changes that could influence quality of life.

Construct validity for the tool in Study 1 was established using a factor analysis technique. Details of this analysis have been reported, but will be summarized here. Three well-defined factors were identified. The most important factor was found to be psychological well-being, followed by physical well-being and symptom control. The fourth factor was a financial factor, which was not useful for the populations tested because they were patients at a medical center where patients receive free care. Psychological well-being included the following items:

general quality of life, fun, satisfaction, usefulness, and sleep. Physical well-being was defined as strength, appetite, work, eating, and sexual functioning. Symptom control included pain, nausea, and vomiting.

Discriminant validity was established by comparing scores for the four groups using analysis of variance to pinpoint differences. As expected, results revealed that the mean score for nonpatients was the highest, indicating the best quality of life. The lowest score was for chemotherapy inpatients. These differences revealed that the instrument was discriminating between groups.

Concurrent validity involved comparisons of scores on the quality of life instrument with scores obtained on physician estimates of quality of life, prognosis, and Karnofsky ratings. The most consistently significant positive correlations were achieved with the physicians' Karnofsky ratings. Although the Karnofsky ratings were useful for measuring performance, they could only account for approximately 29 percent of the variance in QLI. This indicates the need for a patient self-rating of quality of life on a multidimensional index.

A corollary of Study 1 was a comparison of the QLI of 77 diabetic females with the responses of the 48 nonpatients, 43 chemotherapy outpatients, 39 radiation outpatients, and 48 chemotherapy inpatients.[12] Summary scores indicated that the highest (best) mean quality of life score was obtained by the nonpatients, with diabetic outpatients and cancer outpatients scoring similarly (Table 1). The cancer inpatients scored the lowest, illustrating that the instrument was sensitive to the degree of illness in the patient.

In summary, the 14-item QLI provides a reliable and valid multidimensional operational definition of quality of life. The most important dimension of quality of life is psychological well-being, followed by physical well-being and symptom

TABLE 1
Mean and *F* Values for the Overall QLI Score and Subscores of the 14-Item QLI across Four Samples[a]

Score	Non-patients	Diabetic Out-patients	Cancer Out-patients	Cancer Inpatients	*F*	*p*
Psychological well-being	90	68	68	51	29.30	< 0.001
Physical well-being	94	69	64	43	50.23	< 0.001
Symptoms	93	83	85	78	8.55	< 0.001
Overall QLI	91	70	71	55	40.75	< 0.001

[a]The mean scores in this table are calculated in the following manner. The overall QLI score is calculated for each subject as the mean of all the 14-item scores and is then calculated for each sample as the mean of the overall QLI scores across sample subjects. The subscores representing the factors of quality of life are calculated in the same way but include only those items pertaining to the factor. QLI scores represent a response on a 100 mm scale.

Reprinted with permission from M. M. Grant, G. V. Padilla, C. Presant, et al., "Cancer Patients and Quality of Life," *Proceedings of the Fourth National Conference on Cancer Nursing, 1983* (New York: American Cancer Society, 1984).

control. The single item that asks subjects to rate their general quality of life is most closely associated with psychological well-being. This indicates that perceived quality of life is essentially mediated by cognitive processes.

STUDY 2

The next step in the development of this tool was to revise the content, refining some items and adding new ones. Items on sexual satisfaction, eating, and pain were revised so as to be responsive to patients who were comfortable with minimal sexual activity, ate very little, and needed a measurement of frequency and severity of pain. Other items were added to reflect interpersonal and body image aspects of self worth. The instrument was revised for a colostomy patient population. Nine items were added, bringing the total to 23 items (see Fig. 1). A change was made in the format of the instrument. In Study 1, the anchor words used for five items reflected extremes of a subjective state whereas nine items of the instrument used the end points "none and not at all" to "normal for me." The revised tool used extreme subjective states to anchor all 23 items. The sample consisted of 135 subjects, for whom the most common diagnosis was colorectal cancer. Other diagnoses included gynecological cancer, Crohn's disease, and colostomies performed for a variety of other reasons.

Construct validity was again established and, because the tool was revised, included a repeat factor analysis. Six factors were identified. As in Study 1, psychological well-being was found to be the most important dimension of quality of life, followed by physical well-being. The other factors were body image (colostomy) concerns, diagnosis/treatment (surgical) response, diagnosis/treatment (nutritional) response, and social concerns (Table 2). The psychological well-being factor was defined by six items: happiness, satisfaction, fun, general quality of life, pleasure in eating, and sleep. The internal consistency for the subset of items was 0.84. The physical well-being factor was defined by strength, fatigue, ability to work, health, and perceived usefulness. Internal consistency was 0.87. The body image (colostomy) concerns factor was defined by the ability to look at the colostomy, tendency to worry, ability to adjust, and ability to live with the odor pertaining to the colostomy. Internal consistency was 0.80. Next was the diagnosis/treatment (surgical) response factor defined by ability to have sufficient sexual activity and frequency and severity of pain. Internal consistency was 0.71. The fifth factor was diagnosis/treatment (nutritional) response as defined by weight and sufficient eating. Internal consistency was 0.48, the poorest. The sixth factor was labeled social concerns because it was defined by social rejection, social contact, and privacy needs. Internal consistency was 0.90.

Table 3 shows that items reflecting social concerns received the highest quality of life scores, followed by nutrition, colostomy concerns, psychological well-being, surgical responses, and physical well-being.

FIGURE 1
Twenty-Three Item QLI for Colostomy Patients

1. How much strength do you have?

100mm*

  None at all   A great deal

2. Is the amount of time you sleep sufficient to meet your needs?

  Not at all sufficient   Completely sufficient

3. Do you tire easily?

  Not at all   A great deal

4. Do you feel your present weight is a problem?

  Not at all   A great deal

5. Do you feel worried (fearful or anxious) about your colostomy?

  Not at all   A great deal

6. Is your sexual activity sufficient to meet your needs?

  Not at all sufficient   Completely sufficient

7. How is your present state of health?

  Extremely poor   Excellent

8. How easy is it to adjust to your colostomy?

  Not at all easy   Extremely easy

9. How much fun do you have (hobbies, recreation, social activities)?

  None at all   A great deal

10. Do you find eating a pleasure?

  Not at all   A great deal

11. How much can you work at your usual tasks (housework, office work, gardening)?

  Not at all   A great deal

12. Is the amount you eat sufficient to meet your needs?

  Not at all sufficient   Completely sufficient

13. How useful do you feel?

  Not at all   Extremely useful

FIG. 1 (continued)

14. How much happiness do you feel?

———————————————————————————————
None at all   A great deal

15. How satisfying is your life?

———————————————————————————————
Not at all   Extremely satisfying

16. How much pain do you feel?

———————————————————————————————
None   Excruciating

17. How often do you feel pain?

———————————————————————————————
Never   All the time

18. How good is the quality of your life?

———————————————————————————————
Extremely poor   Excellent

19. How fearful are you of odor or leakage from your colostomy?

———————————————————————————————
Not at all   Extremely fearful

20. Is your level of contact with your friends and family sufficient to meet your needs?

———————————————————————————————
Not at all sufficient   Completely sufficient

21. Do you feel rejected by your family or loved ones?

———————————————————————————————
Not at all   Extremely

22. How difficult is it for you to look at your colostomy?

———————————————————————————————
Not at all difficult   Extremely

23. Is the amount of privacy you have sufficient to meet your needs?

———————————————————————————————
Not at all sufficient   Completely sufficient

*Length of scale.

Reprinted with permission from M. M. Grant, G. V. Padilla, C. Presant, et al., "Cancer Patients and Quality of Life," *Proceedings of the Fourth National Conference on Cancer Nursing, 1983* (New York: American Cancer Society, 1984).

TABLE 2
Rotated Factor Loadings with Orthogonal Varimax Method for Items in the QLI for Colostomy Patients (*n* = 82)[a]

Items	Psychological Well-Being	Physical Well-Being	Body Image (Colostomy) Concerns	Diagnosis/ Treatment (Surgical) Response	Diagnosis/ Treatment (Nutritional) Response	Social Concerns
Happiness	0.82					
Satisfaction	0.80					
Fun	0.75					
General quality of life	0.71			0.34		
Pleasure in eating	0.53		0.30			
Sleep	0.41				0.31	
Strength		0.80				
Fatigue		0.75			0.40	
Work	0.54	0.71				
Health	0.37	0.70				
Usefulness	0.40	0.65				
Worry, colostomy			0.83			
Look, colostomy			0.79			
Adjust, colostomy			0.76			
Fear odor			0.69			
Sexual functioning				0.67		
Pain, frequency		0.56		0.65		
Pain, intensity		0.54		0.58		
Weight				0.35	0.74	
Eating, sufficient					0.71	
Social rejection						0.79
Social contact					0.33	0.71
Privacy				0.36		0.57

[a]All loadings of 0.25 or less are omitted.

TABLE 3
Mean Values for the Overall QLI Score and Subscores of the
23-Item QLI for Colostomy Patients[a]

Score	Number of Patients	Mean
Psychological well-being	132	61.0
Physical well-being	134	45.0
Body image (colostomy) concerns	126	69.5
Diagnosis/treatment (surgical) response	94	59.5
Diagnosis/treatment (nutritional) response	133	73.5
Social concerns	134	83.5
Overall QLI	134	61.0

[a]The mean scores in this table are calculated in the following manner. The overall QLI is calculated for each subject as the mean of all the 23-item scores, and the subscores representing the factors of quality of life are calculated in the same manner but include only those items pertaining to the factor. QLI scores represent a response on a 100 mm scale.

To compare the results of the 23-item QLI with that obtained from the previous 14-item QLI, and to further establish discriminant validity, mean scores were calculated using items common to both instruments (Table 4). Results revealed that the nonpatients had the highest mean score, the inpatients had the lowest scores, diabetics and outpatients fell in the middle, and the colostomy patients had the second to the poorest score. In the revised form, the instrument was still discriminating sick subjects from well subjects. The colostomy patients rated their quality of life approximately one week after discharge from the hospital. They were comparable to other outpatient populations inasmuch as they were no longer in the hospital. Yet they had lower quality of life scores than the other two outpatient populations. It seems that the impact on quality of life is greater for patients who have colostomies and are recently discharged from the hospital than for either radiation outpatients or chemotherapy outpatients.

DISCUSSION OF STUDY 1 AND STUDY 2

Interpretation of the results of Studies 1 and 2 can be made by examining the findings in light of Flanagan's work on quality of life for the general population.[13] Flanagan analyzed a total of 6,500 critical incidents submitted in response to questions about what incidents had a significant positive or negative effect on overall quality of life. Fifteen factors were identified by several independent judges, and included virtually all of the 6,500 incidents. Factors were then ranked by 1,000 30-year-olds, 1,000 50-year-olds, and 1,000 70-year-olds in relation to the question "What is your overall quality of life at the present time?"

TABLE 4
Quality of Life Mean Scores Based on 11 Comparable Items[a]

	Number of Subjects	Mean Score
Nonpatients	48	91
Diabetics	77	69
Outpatients:		
Chemotherapy	42	70
Radiation	39	60
Colostomy	70	57
Inpatients:		
Chemotherapy	48	52

[a]The mean scores in this table are calculated in the following manner. Using only items common to all samples, the score is calculated for each subject as the mean of all item scores and is then calculated for each sample as the mean of the average score across sample subjects. Scores represent a response on a 100 mm scale.

Reprinted with permission from M. M. Grant, G. V. Padilla, C. Presant, et al., "Cancer Patients and Quality of Life," *Proceedings of the Fourth National Conference on Cancer Nursing, 1983* (New York: American Cancer Society, 1984).

The items most closely associated with quality of life were material comfort, work, health, active recreation, learning, close relationship with spouse, and socializing, in that order. Some of these factors are dealt with in programs for cancer patients, such as "I Can Cope," and "Can Surmount." The reason these programs enjoy success with cancer patients may be that they provide recreation, learning, close relationships, and socialization.

Apparently other aspects of quality of life of cancer patients are not being as well addressed. Psychological well-being, surgical response, and especially physical well-being subscores are consistently lower than the other scores and reveal the need for more help for the patients' physical well-being.

In summary, the 23-item QLI again provides support for a multidimensional operational definition of quality of life. As in Study 1, the most important dimension of quality of life continues to be psychological well-being, followed by physical well-being, body image (colostomy) concerns, responses to diagnosis/treatments (surgical, nutritional), and social concerns. As in Study 1, the single item on the tool about general quality of life is most closely associated with psychological well-being. This finding further supports the notion that quality of life is essentially predicted by cognitive processes. Findings across several studies establish the initial reliability and validity of a multidimensional tool.

A CONCEPTUAL MODEL FOR QUALITY OF LIFE AS AN OUTCOME VARIABLE

Burckhardt provides important insight into the use of quality of life as an outcome variable in explaining that quality of life is mediated by cognitive variables such as perceived support, negative attitude toward illness, self-esteem, and internal control over health.[14] The findings suggest that manipulating input variables such as pain or impairment may not directly impact on quality of life as one might intuitively predict. Rather, these input variables impact on cognitive mediating variables such as self-esteem and perceived control over health that, in turn, are directly related to changes in quality of life. Not surprisingly, Studies 1 and 2 reported above indicate that the cognitive-emotional dimension, psychological well-being, is the most important predictor of quality of life. A related cognitive-emotional dimension, body image concerns, is also important.

In addition to Burckhardt's study, those of Grant et al., Lewis, Padilla et al., and Young and Longman affirm the significance of perceived self-worth (self-esteem, usefulness) in promoting quality of life, particularly within the context of psychological well-being.[15] Self-worth can be affected by perceived personal control over health and activities by the nurse that are perceived to affirm self-worth. However, there should also be a differential impact on different dimensions of quality of life. Perceived personal control over health should form a greater correlation with physical well-being and response to diagnosis/treatment (symptom control) factors of quality of life, whereas perceived nurse activities that affirm patient worth should correlate more highly with psychological well-being, body image concerns, and social concerns.

Although Burckhardt's research successfully used a composite single score to measure quality of life, her findings indicate that a multidimensional quality of life construct would be more useful in measuring the impact of nursing process on quality of life outcome. Quality of life of patients, that which makes life worth living for an ill person, is affected by numerous factors over which nursing has little or no control. These are factors such as diagnosis, family illness history, predisposing characteristics, and medical treatment. Quality of life is also affected by factors over which nursing may in fact exercise a significant amount of control. These factors may include environmental, informational, personal, or social type variables as well as nursing treatment. A multidimensional, operational definition of quality of life, one that measures psychological well-being, physical well-being, body image concerns, response to diagnosis/treatment, and social concerns, can measure both the direct and indirect effects of nursing process along with the effects of nonnursing variables.

Figure 2 provides a model of the concept of how the research construct, quality of life, works as a nursing care outcome variable. The model is based on Study 2, in which the impact was examined of a quality assurance program for cancer nursing on various patient outcomes including quality of life, as well as on the studies of Burckhardt and Lewis.[16]

The independent variable, the variable manipulated by the investigator, may include nursing process activities that impact directly on specific dimensions of quality of life, such as care of the colostomy that impacts on physical well-being.

FIGURE 2
A Model of the Relationship between Nursing Process and the Dimensions of Quality of Life

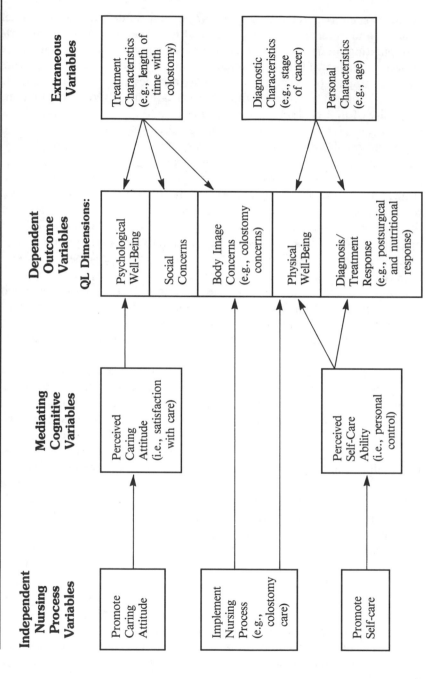

The impact of other nursing process variables, such as promotion of self-care in the patient and a caring attitude on the part of the nurse regarding quality of life, is mediated by cognitive activity. The mediating variable is a necessary antecedent to quality of life. For that reason, nursing process has an indirect impact on quality of life. For example, promotion of self-care must result in perceived ability to care for self that may be measured as personal control. Another example is promotion of a caring attitude that must be perceived by the patient and can be measured as satisfaction with nursing activities. Both caring activities and personal control act to affirm self-worth and for that reason impact on quality of life. It is expected that perceived personal control over illness impacts primarily on physical well-being, although satisfaction with care that affirms patient worth impacts primarily on psychological well-being. A single quality of life score is unlikely to be a sensitive measure of various types of nursing activities. In addition, failure to take into account cognitive mediating variables may make it difficult to interpret findings, especially in the event that the nursing activity fails to result in a change in quality of life.

Thus the model predicts that some nursing interventions, seen as manipulated independent variables, produce cognitive-emotional changes in the patient that enhance perceptions of self-worth. Self-worth is the necessary cognitive-emotional mediator to produce psychological well-being, the central most significant dimension of quality of life.

Control over health or illness-related events is strongly valued and has been shown to have positive effects.[17] Perceptions of control over illness may reduce feelings of helplessness, thereby promoting recovery.[18] Actual control over daily activities may improve alertness, physical health, and psychological well-being,[19] as well as morale.[20] Perceived personal control is measured using the Multidimensional Health Locus of Control Scale that has published reliability and validity.[21]

Satisfaction with nursing care is measured using a revised form of a tool developed by Ware et al.[22] It was originally a 43-item questionnaire that has been pared to a 32-item tool. The tool has construct validity. A factor analysis of the responses of 81 patients with colostomies yielded a six-factor construct consisting of the following dimensions. The most important dimensions that affirm patient worth are nurse availability and confidence in nursing care. The six items defining nurse availability have an alpha coefficient of 0.90; the seven items defining confidence in nursing care yield an alpha coefficient of 0.78. The items that define nurse availability focus on nurse response to the patient, such as no waiting, responding to call light, helping with pain, not making patients feel foolish, helping with patient questions, and anticipating patient needs. Those that define confidence in the nurse include: nurses keep patient from worrying, do not take risks, explain things, provide individualized care, and other items.

Extraneous variables are those that impact on outcomes but are not manipulated by the investigator. Extraneous variables are usually controlled either directly or statistically. They may include diagnostic characteristics such as stage of cancer, treatment characteristics such as length of time with colostomy, and personal characteristics such as age. Information on stage of cancer and age was obtained from the medical record. Stage of cancer and age are expected to have a significant negative correlation with physical well-being and diagnosis/treatment response, whereas length of time with colostomy is expected to correlate positively with psychological well-being, body image concerns, and social concerns.

RESULTS

One hundred thirty-five patients with colostomies (Study 2) filled out the Satisfaction with Nursing Care tool and the Multidimensional Health Locus of Control Scale. Table 5 provides the correlations between the overall QLI score and subscores and the satisfaction scores, i.e., personal control, stage of cancer, age, and length of time with colostomy. In accordance with with the stated predictions based on the model diagramed in Figure 2, satisfaction with nursing care as measured by nurse availability was positively and most significantly correlated with psychological well-being. It is correlated significantly with social concerns and physical well-being. Confidence in the nurse correlated most significantly with both psychological well-being and social concerns. It also correlated significantly but to a lesser degree with all the other quality of life scores.

In terms of perceived control, it was expected that increased perceived control would be correlated with increased psychological well-being. The results from the chance locus of control score supported the prediction. As chance decreased (control increases) as a perceived cause of illness-wellness, physical well-being increased. The negative correlation between chance and physical well-being was the most significant; however, chance also correlated significantly with overall QLI and psychological well-being.

A third prediction was that age and stage of cancer would correlate negatively with physical well-being and diagnosis/treatment response. In fact, the negative correlations between stage of cancer and physical well-being and one of the diagnosis/treatment response variables were the strongest, although minimally significant. With respect to age, the negative correlation with the other diagnosis/treatment response variable was the strongest and most significant. However, no significant correlation was found between age and physical well-being.

Finally, it was expected that increased length of time with colostomy would be positively correlated with increased psychological well-being and increased quality of life in terms of body image concerns and social concerns. Only the correlation with social concerns was significant, but in the opposite direction to that which was predicted. As length of time with the colostomy increased, quality of life with respect to social concerns deteriorated.

Of the eight correlations possible with the overall QLI score, three (37.5%) were significant in the direction congruent with the model: i.e., as confidence in the nurse increased, internality increased, and chance decreased as an illness-

TABLE 5
Correlations between QLI Overall and Subscores, and Satisfaction with Care, Personal Control, and Extraneous Variables ($n = 120\text{-}135$)

Cognitive-Emotional Mediating Variables	Rotated Factor Loadings						
	Overall QLI	Psychological Well-Being	Physical Well-Being	Body Image (Colostomy) Concerns	Diagnosis/ Treatment (Surgical) Response	Diagnosis/ Treatment (Nutritional) Response	Social Concerns
Satisfaction with care							
Availability of RN	0.13	0.30[a]	0.25[a]	0.12	0.09	0.20[a]	0.27[a]
Confidence in RN	0.31[a]	0.37[a]	0.21[a]	0.25[a]	0.20[a]	0.23[a]	0.38[a]
Personal control							
Internality	0.20[a]	0.17	0.16	0.18	0.18	0.03	0.05
Chance	- 0.27[a]	- 0.28[a]	- 0.35[a]	- 0.19	- 0.18	- 0.17	- 0.06
Powerful other	0.07	- 0.07	0.09	0.04	0.08	0.06	- 0.13
Extraneous variables							
Stage of cancer	0.02	- 0.03	- 0.18	0.11	0.03	- 0.20[a]	0.14
Age	0.21[a]	- 0.01	0.04	0.19	0.31[a]	0.06	0.12
Length of time with colostomy	- 0.09	- 11	- 0.003	0.06	- 0.14	- 0.04	- 0.23[a]

[a] The critical values of r for a two-tailed test of a when df ≥ 100 are $r = .195$ for $p \leq .05$, and $r = .254$ for $p \leq .01$. E. S. Pearson and H. O. Hartley, *Biometrika Tables for Statisticians*, Vol. 1 (New York: Cambridge University Press, 1962), p. 138.

wellness cause, then overall quality of life increased. Of the 13 predictions made for the various quality of life dimensions, five (38%) were supported. These findings provide only beginning support for the conceptual model of the way in which quality of life works as a multidimensional outcome variable. It is appealing and has potential. Inasmuch as the model was superimposed, a posteriori, on the data, it is not surprising that the results were weak. Future prospective research is needed to test the model. Is quality of life a multidimensional construct that may be directly or indirectly impacted by the nursing process? Do nursing interventions that improve self-worth also promote psychological well-being within the context of quality of life? Is self-worth a necessary cognitive-emotional mediator that produces psychological well-being? Is psychological well-being the most significant dimension of quality of life? Findings on "confidence in the RN" as a subset of the Satisfaction with Care Tool show positive and significant correlations with all the QLI factors. Thus, a promising area for future research would take the kinds of activities that define "confidence in the RN" and manipulate them as independent variables in an experimental design.

ABOUT THE AUTHORS

At the time of writing, Geraldine V. Padilla, PhD, was Director, and Marcia M. Grant, MSN, RN, was Assistant Director, Department of Nursing Research, City of Hope Medical Center, Duarte, California.

REFERENCES

1. F. Baker and J. Intagliata, "Quality of Life in the Evaluation of Community Support Systems," *Evaluation Program Planning,* 5 (1982), 69–79.

2. J. M. Laborde and M. J. Powers, "Satisfaction with Life for Patients Undergoing Hemodialysis and Patients Suffering from Osteoarthritis," *Research in Nursing & Health,* 3 (1980), 19–24.

3. K. J. Young and A. J. Longman, "Quality of Life and Persons with Melanoma: A Pilot Study," *Cancer Nursing,* 6 (1983), 219–225.

4. F. M. Lewis, "Experienced Personal Control and Quality of Life in Late Stage Cancer Patients," *Nursing Research,* 31 (1982), 113–119.

5. C. S. Burckhardt, "The Impact of Arthritis on Quality of Life," *Nursing Research,* 34(1) (1984), 11–16.

6. A. Grieco and C. L. Long, "Investigation of the Karnofsky Performance Status as a Measure of Quality of Life," *Health Psychology,* 3 (1984), 129–142.

7. D. Karnofsky and J. Burchenal, "The Clinical Evaluation of Chemotherapeutic Agents in Cancer," in C. M. MacLeod, ed., *Evaluation of Chemotherapeutic Agents* (New York: Columbia Press, 1949).

8. I. R. Gough, C. M. Furnival, L. Schilder, et al., "Assessment of the Quality of Life of Patients with Advanced Cancer," *European Journal of Cancer & Clinical Oncology,* 19 (1983), 1161–1165.

9. C. A. Presant, C. Klahr, and L. Hogan, "Evaluating Quality of Life in Oncology Patients: Pilot Observations," *Oncology Nursing Forum,* 8(3) (1981), 26–30.

10. G. V. Padilla, C. Presant, M. Grant, et al., "Quality of Life Index for Patients with Cancer," *Research in Nursing & Health,* 6 (1983), 117–126.

11. Ibid.

12. M. M. Grant, G. V. Padilla, C. Presant, et al., "Cancer Patients and Quality of Life," *Proceedings of the Fourth National Conference on Cancer Nursing, 1983* (New York: American Cancer Society, 1984), 2–11.

13. J. C. Flanagan, "Measurement of Quality of Life: Current State of the Art," *Archives of Physical Medicine & Rehabilitation,* 63 (1982), 56–59.

14. Burckhardt, "The Impact of Arthritis on Quality of Life."

15. Grant, Padilla, Presant, et al., "Cancer Patients and Quality of Life"; Lewis, "Experienced Personal Control and Quality of Life in Late Stage Cancer Patients"; Padilla, Presant, Grant, et al., "Quality of Life Index for Patients with Cancer"; and Young and Longman, "Quality of Life and Persons with Melanoma."

16. Burckhardt, "The Impact of Arthritis on Quality of Life"; and Lewis, "Experienced Personal Control and Quality of Life in Late Stage Cancer Patients."

17. L. S. Linn and C. E. Lewis, "Attitudes toward Self-Care among Practicing Physicians," *Medical Care,* 17 (1979), 183–190.

18. D. S. Krantz and R. Schulz, "A Model of Life Crisis, Control, and Health Outcomes: Cardiac Rehabilitation and Relocation of the Elderly," in A. Baum and J. E. Singer, eds., *Advances in Environmental Psychology* (Hillsdale, NJ: Lawrence Erlbaum, 1980).

19. J. Rodin and E. Langer, "Long-Term Effects of a Control-Relevant Intervention with Institutionalized Aged," *Journal of Personality and Social Psychology,* 35 (1977), 897–902; and R. Schulz, "Aging and Control," in J. Garber and M. E. P. Seligman, eds., *Human Helplessness: Theory and Application* (New York: Academic Press, 1980).

20. B. L. Chang, "Perceived Situational Control of Daily Activities: A New Tool," *Research in Nursing and Health,* 1 (1978), 181–188.

21. K. A. Wallston, B. S. Wallston, and R. DeVellis, "Development of the Multidimensional Health Locus of Control (MHLC) Scales," *Health Education Monographs,* 6 (1978), 160–170.

22. J. E. Ware, M. K. Snyder, and W. R. Wright, *Development and Validation of Scales to Measure Patient Satisfaction with Health Care Services,* Final Report, Vol. 1, Part A: "Review of Literature, Overview of Methods, and Results Regarding Construction of Scales"; Part B: "Results Regarding Scales Constructed from the Patient Satisfaction Questionnaire and Measures of Other Health Care Perceptions" (Carbondale: Southern Illinois University School of Medicine, 1976).

Quality Assurance Manual of the Home Care Association of Washington

Bernadette Lalonde

The reprint presented here consists of selected excerpts from the first edition of the Quality Assurance Manual of the Home Care Association of Washington. *The project described in the section on Manual Purposes is the first federally supported research effort to rigorously identify outcomes applicable to a wide range of home care recipients. Thus, the project's significance is enhanced by its potential contribution to public policy discussions regarding the effectiveness of home care.*

The second section excerpted from the manual, addressing reliability and validity, is included to provide general background in evaluating outcomes presented throughout this volume. Although the excerpt is a brief review of the concepts of reliability and validity, it serves as a reminder that to adequately define valid outcomes is a challenge for any health provider.

Finally, the entire chapter on one of the outcome measures, discharge status, is reprinted in full with grateful acknowledgement to Dr. Lalonde

Excerpted with permission of Bernadette Lalonde and the Home Care Association of Washington from Bernadette Lalonde, *Quality Assurance Manual of the Home Care Association of Washington* (Edmonds, WA: Home Care Association of Washington, July 1986), copyright © 1986, Home Care Association of Washington.

The research described here was supported by the Health Care Financing Administration under Cooperative Agreement Number 18-C-98868/0-01. The opinions expressed herein are those of the author and should not be construed to represent the views or policies of any agency of the United States government.

and the Home Care Association of Washington. The excerpt provides a comprehensive description of one outcome tool and its use. Although each tool in the manual varies considerably in format and data collection requirements, this excerpt offers the reader an excellent sample of the breadth and depth of the Home Care Association of Washington's project and the quality of work it is producing.

INTRODUCTION

Manual Purpose

Initially, this manual was intended to be the vehicle by which the Home Care Association of Washington would share the research findings of a three-year grant (1985-1988) funded by the Health Care Financing Administration (HCFA). The grant—at the end of its first year at the time of this writing—was to develop, pilot test, and refine a total of seven reliable and valid outcome scales for the home care industry. However, as the Quality Assurance Committee of the Home Care Association of Washington fully intends to continue its work developing and testing quality assurance scales for the home care industry past the life of the HCFA grant, the manual has evolved to be the mechanism by which the Home Care Association of Washington's Quality Assurance Committee will share its continued work in the area of quality assurance. In addition to sharing this work with the Home Care Association of Washington's membership, the manual is available to other interested parties. It is anticipated the manual will prove useful to any individual or agency providing or researching long term care for the elderly. The manual is expected to prove particularly beneficial to other home care agencies across the nation and to hospice agencies.

The first edition of the manual presents three of the seven outcome scales developed in the first year of the HCFA grant: General Symptom Distress, Discharge Status, and Taking Medications as Prescribed. The second and third editions will house the remaining scales developed and tested in the course of the HCFA grant, as well as other quality assurance scales developed apart from the grant (e.g., a client satisfaction survey for home care, a utilization review scale). Subsequently developed and tested scales will be made available to holders of earlier editions of the manual upon request.[1]

The Method Used to Develop and Test the Scales in this Manual

The scales in the manual were developed via a particular method to ensure they were:

- Tailored to home care's unique characteristics.

- Acceptable to home care staff and administrators.
- Reliable and valid.
- Feasible and cost-effective.

To ensure the outcome scales were tailored to home care's unique characteristics and acceptable to home care staff and administrators, the Home Care Association of Washington's Quality Assurance Committee (hereafter referred to as the Committee) worked in close collaboration with the principal investigator of the HCFA grant, Dr. Bernadette Lalonde, to develop the scales. The Committee was comprised of a member of the Home Care Association of Washington's Board of Directors and fourteen home care agency directors and/or direct service providers from home care agencies across Washington state. The Committee met with the principal investigator once a month and was actively involved in all steps of scale development and testing. The Committee and their agencies' staff were responsible for:

1. Rating the appropriateness and importance of an extensive list of possible outcome criteria for which scales could be developed.
2. Ranking the criteria and, in essence, choosing which criteria should be addressed in each year of the three year HCFA grant.
3. Determining the discharge locations and primary reasons for discharge which comprise the Discharge Status Scale.
4. Determining the general symptoms which appear on the General Symptom Distress Scale as well as the scoring system for this scale.
5. Determining the questions which needed to be asked on the medications scale as well as the scale's scoring system.
6. Helping to develop precise instructions on how to implement and score each scale.

To test the reliability and validity of the scales, the scales were pilot tested in each of five home care agencies across the state of Washington. The data were computer analyzed and the scales found to be reliable and valid. Evidence of reliability and validity is presented under each outcome chapter. In addition, the scales were evaluated—by each pilot test agency's staff—in terms of (a) their appropriateness to home care, (b) the completeness of each scale, (c) final scoring categories, (d) ease of understanding and (e) ease to complete. The scales and their instructions were modified per this feedback.

To ensure the feasibility and cost-effectiveness of the scales, each scale was kept short and succinct. The time to complete each scale was tested during the pilot testing of the scales. On average, they require between two and ten minutes to complete.

Notes on Reliability and Validity

Reliability. Reliability indicates the extent to which individual differences in scale scores are attributable to "true" differences in the characteristics under consideration and the extent to which they are attributable to chance errors or irrelevancies (e.g., weather, excess noise in the environment at the time of assessment, the mood of the client when filling out a satisfaction survey, the instructions given or questions asked to determine the extent of the client's medication knowledge, rapport between the client and examiner). Hence, one strives to control the irrelevancies which might affect scales scores. The crux of the matter, of course, lies in the definition of error variance/irrelevancies. Factors that might be considered error variance for one purpose might be classified under true variance for another. For example, if we are interested in measuring fluctuations of mood, then the day-by-day changes in scores on a depression scale would be relevant to the purpose of the scale and would be part of the true variance of the scores. If, on the other hand, the scale is designed to measure client knowledge, fluctuations in mood would fall under the heading of error variance. Essentially, any condition that is irrelevant to the purpose of the scale represents error variance. Thus, when one tries to maintain uniform administration conditions by standardizing the instructions or questions asked, by explicitly stating what constitutes a knowledgeable and unknowledgeable response, by using the same method to collect the information, one is reducing error variance and making scale scores more reliable. Despite optimum testing conditions, however, no scale is a perfectly reliable instrument. Hence, every scale should be accompanied by a statement of its reliability.

There could, of course, be as many varieties of scale reliability as there are conditions affecting scale scores. In actual practice, however, the types of reliability computed are relatively few. They are as follows.

Interrater Reliability: This measures the level of accuracy with which two or more people document or score the observation made. This is an important reliability coefficient when observer judgment is necessary. One controls for this error, in part, by standardizing scoring instructions and training staff. One assesses interrater reliability by having two or more observers score the same client's chart or the client's responses to a particular interview question. Interrater reliability is usually expressed as a percent agreement or correlation coefficient. Acceptable interrater reliability is usually set at 80-100 percent.

Test-Retest Reliability: This type of reliability measures the stability of the scale over time, and is tested when one believes that the characteristic of interest should not change over time (e.g., IQ). Hence, this type of reliability test is not appropriate to all scales. It measures the degree of association between sets of measurements collected at two or more points in time. The degree of association is expressed as a zero-order coefficient (e.g., Pearson product-moment correlation coefficient, Spearman rank order coefficient).

Internal Consistency Reliability: This type of reliability examines the intercorrelations or covariance of all individual items making up a scale. It is tested on a multi-item scale (e.g., an 18-item patient satisfaction survey) when one believes that the multi-item scale represents only one aspect of the characteristic of interest. The higher the intercorrelations among the items, the greater is the scale's internal consistency reliability.

Validity. The validity of a scale represents the extent to which the scale adequately measures the concepts under study. It reflects the extent to which the scale correctly measures the characteristic studied. The principal validity categories follow.

Content Validity: Content validity indicates the extent to which the instrument has adequately sampled the behavior domain to be measured. It is built into a scale from the onset through the choice of appropriate items. To do this, one systematically examines relevant information on the characteristic to be measured, lists items to be included in the scale, and has experts rate each item for its appropriateness.

Face Validity: This type of validity is judged by external experts who logically determine if the scale "looks like" what it is supposed to measure. It measures whether the scale looks relevant and appropriate to the experts in the field who may be using the scale.

Construct Validity: Construct validity confirms or disconfirms a priori assumptions about relationships among variables (e.g., effects of demographic variables on the characteristic of interest). It is tested by specifying—before analyses are done—relationships you would expect to find or not find. For example, one a priori hypothesis regarding a symptom distress scale might be that one would expect clients with a primary diagnosis of cancer to report more nausea/vomiting problems than would clients with a primary diagnosis of congestive heart failure.

DISCHARGE STATUS

Scale Purpose

This scale (see Fig. 1) is intended to augment individual agencies' discharge summary forms. As the possible discharge location and primary discharge reason options are clearly delineated, the scale enables staff to begin to document this information consistently and reliably. Used in combination with the Discharge Status Score Summary, it provides agencies a quick overview of their discharge activity.

FIGURE 1
Discharge Status Scale

Client's Chart Number _____

Length of Stay Last Admission _____ Days

Primary Diagnosis _____

DISCHARGE STATUS

DISCHARGE LOCATION   LOCATION [ ]

Client's Own Home
1. Lives alone, without referral to other community resources
2. Lives alone with referral
3. Lives with others in own home, without referral to other community resources
4. Lives with others in own home, with referral

Family Member's Home
5. Without referral to other community resources
6. With referral

Foster Care/Adult Family Home
7. Without referral to other community resources
8. With referral

Congregate Care/Retirement Facility
9. Without referral to other community resources
10. With referral

11. Nursing Home
12. Acute Care Hospital
13. Psychiatric Hospital/Inpatient Substance Abuse Treatment/Certified Rehab Unit

Expired
14. At home
15. In health care facility

16. OTHER (Specify: _____
_____
_____

PRIMARY REASON FOR DISCHARGE   PRIMARY REASON [ ]

1. No longer meets homebound regulations as specified by Medicare or other third party payors.
2. Client no longer requires any skilled care.
3. Client/family requires skilled care but client/family can manage alone.
4. Client/family refused service.
5. Admitted to health care facility.
6. Requires type of service not provided.
7. Agency has insufficient resources.
8. Client/family has insufficient financial resources.
9. Continued care not approved or authorized by physician.
10. Continued/prolonged noncompliance on part of client/family.
11. Moved out of agency service area.
12. Expired
13. OTHER (Please Specify) _____

Completion

Who May Complete. Following training, this form may be completed by clerical/records staff or the client's professional caregiver.

Training Staff to Complete the Scale. To ensure all staff within your agency are completing the scale the same way, it is recommended that all staff expected to complete the scale be trained. Ensure that staff know how to complete the scale and they know the distinctions between each of the discharge location options and each of the discharge reasons.

In training, it is recommended that each staff person be given five to ten randomly selected clients' charts and have them independently complete a scale for each chart. Have at least one professional staff person also complete a scale for each of the same five to ten charts. This should be done independently and without knowledge of how the other staff scored the scales. Compare the two sets of scores for each chart. If there are differences, it will be necessary to discuss the differences with the two staff persons involved and to resolve the differences. Clear, explicitly stated policy decisions may need to be made concerning what is to be considered the correct discharge location or *primary* reason for discharge if discrepancies in scores continue.

It is very important that all staff expected to complete the scale be trained sufficiently to ensure that if all of them completed Discharge Status Scales on the same charts, they would have assigned the same scores *at least* 85 percent of the time. This will ensure the interrater reliability of your scores and allow you to say with confidence that differences in obtained scores represent "true" differences in discharge location and discharge reason and not differences between staff interpretations of the discharge summary notes in the charts.

When to Complete. The scale is intended to be completed following the client's complete discharge from the home care agency. It is not intended for completion following termination of each home care service (e.g., RN, OT, PT, RT, Home Health Aide, etc.). The scale takes approximately two minutes to complete.

At this time, as a standard discharge policy is not employed across home care agencies, each agency should ensure that their discharge policy is clear, precise, and made explicit to all staff. If this is not done, the discharge status information may not be collected uniformly. For example, if your agency does not discharge a client when he/she goes into the hospital and the client dies while in the hospital, it may be your policy to discharge the client at this point (which means that the discharge location will be *15—expired in a health care facility*), or to back date the client's discharge to the last billing date (which means that the discharge location will be *12—acute care hospital*). If this policy is not explicitly stated and clearly understood, your staff will not be collecting your data uniformly or reliably.

As the scale takes such a short time to complete, it is recommended this form be completed on all clients following their discharge from home care and that the form be placed in the client's chart with your agency's discharge summary forms. Thus the data would be readily available for quality assurance review.

Discharge Location Instructions. Following are specific instructions which will help your staff determine the correct discharge location score. Enter the number corresponding to the client's discharge location in the box provided on the Discharge Status scale. This refers to the place where the individual is to be located *following discharge or referral* from home care.

Client's Own Home. If a client owns or is renting a house or apartment alone or with someone (including a family member or live-in), consider it to be the client's own home. Discharge location will be either 1, 2, 3 or 4. See notes on Referral to Other Community Resources for examples of community resources.

With Referral to Other Community Resources. Includes referrals for chore service, meals, live-in, adult day care, volunteer services, health maintenance, private duty nursing or aid service, information and assistance, elderly services, and any outpatient therapies.

Family Member's Home. If the client is *living with a family member in the family member's home,* the client's discharge location will be either 5 or 6. If the client is living in a family member's home without a family member in residence, consider the client to be living in his/her own home. Discharge location will be either 1, 2, 3 or 4.

Foster Care/Adult Family Home. Client is considered discharged to this location if the Adult Family Home or Foster Care is in a private home where the client is given constant supervision. Adult Family Home or Foster Care locations will usually be licensed for six to eight people only.

Congregate Care/Retirement Facility. Can usually house more than eight persons. Client is independent and has own room or apartment. Facility usually provides chore service, meals, some nursing and supervision.

Acute Care Hospital. Does not include a psychiatric hospital or discharge to an inpatient substance abuse treatment center or certified rehab unit. See note on psychiatric hospital.

Psychiatric Hospital/Inpatient Substance Abuse Treatment/Certified Rehab Unit. Includes inpatient alcohol treatment programs. If a client, however, is admitted for an involuntary psychiatric stay in a general hospital, the client would be considered discharged to an acute care hospital.

Expired. Client is to be given the discharge of expired at home if he/she is still on your caseload and actually dies at his/her own home, or a family member's home. If you referred the client to an acute care hospital but did not discharge them, and the client died in hospital they would be considered *15—expired in a health care facility.* If you discharged the client at the point when they entered an acute care hospital and he/she died in the hospital, the discharge location would be *12—acute care hospital.*

Some agencies' discharge policies will preclude them from ever having a score of 15. For example, some agencies do not discharge their clients when they go into the hospital. If the client dies while in the hospital, they back date the client's discharge to the last billing date. This means the client's discharge summary will state the client was discharged to an acute care hospital.

Other. If patient was discharged to a location not listed, please specify location.

Instructions for Primary Reason for Discharge.
Put the number of the *primary* reason in the box. The following notes will help you determine the correct response. It is thought that the response categories are mutually exclusive, but if you should find you are unable to make a firm choice of the *primary* reason between two possible discharge reasons, the agency should make a policy decision on which is to be considered the primary reason. For example, if both 1 and 2 are noted in the client's discharge summary (respectively, "the client no longer meets homebound regulations," and "the client no longer requires any skilled care"), it is likely that most agencies' policies will state that "no longer requires any skilled care" is to be considered the primary reason for discharge.

Client Requires Skilled Care but Client/Family Can Manage Alone. The client is homebound, still requires skilled care, but the family can provide the care instead of home care.

Client/Family Refused Service. The client is homebound, still requires skilled care, but the client and/or family refused service.

Admitted to Health Care Facility. This includes admissions to nursing homes, acute care hospitals, and psychiatric hospital/inpatient substance abuse treatment/certified rehab units.

Requires Type of Service Not Provided. If the admitted client deteriorates or gets better to the point of only requiring a PT, OT, ST, or MSW but the certified agency does not have such a person on staff, this would be the reason for discharge. In essence, this is the reason for discharge if the client now requires a skilled service not provided by the agency.

Agency Has Insufficient Resources. This would be the reason for discharge, for example, if the admitted client now needs only a PT, and the agency's one PT already has a full case load. This would also be the reason for discharge if the client's coverage lapses and the agency was helping with finances of their own, but the agency's financial resources are now depleted. In essence, this would be the reason for discharge if the agency *could usually provide* the required service, but can no longer do it because of staffing shortages or agency financial problems.

Client/Family Has Insufficient Financial Resources. This would be the reason for discharge if the client/family has no fiscal coverage; i.e., they had limited insurance but it has now run out and they cannot pay for continued service, if their coupons were discontinued, or if they were initially on Medicare but are not now.

Continued Care Not Approved or Authorized by Physician. If the client is still homebound and requires skilled service but the physician will not approve further visits nor authorize continued care, this would be the reason for discharge. This would also be the primary reason for discharge if the client refuses to obtain a physician.

Continued/Prolonged Noncompliance on Part of Client/Family. The client is homebound, still requires skilled care but the client and/or family are continually noncompliant.

Moved Out of Agency Service Area. This specifically means the client moved out of your service area. This includes if the client was visiting in your service area, was admitted to your service, and was then discharged because they moved out of your area while they still required skilled care.

Other. If a client is discharged for a reason not listed, please specify the reason. For example, if a husband is being seen by your agency while his wife is being seen by a different home care agency, you may discharge the husband so that both husband and wife are seen by the same home care agency.

Documenting the Time Required to Complete the Scale. During the pilot tests on this scale, it was established that the scale required, on average, two minutes to complete. Agencies, however, may choose to check this out for themselves by asking staff to record the time taken to complete each scale.

Filling in the Client's Chart Number, Diagnosis and Length of Stay. With the exception of the client's chart number, filling in this information on each client's Discharge Status form is optional. It was thought, however, that this data may prove useful to your Quality Assurance Committee when they make some interpretations about the discharge status data you collect.

A number of factors may affect client outcomes: primary diagnosis, living arrangements, length of stay on your service, intensity of care required while on your service, number of complicating diagnoses. In order to make some determination about the appropriateness of discharge locations achieved by your agency, your Quality Assurance Committee will need to take some of these factors into account.

A Demographic Sheet, listing some of the factors which may affect client outcomes, is included under the General Symptom Distress chapter of the complete manual. Agencies may choose to collect all or part of these data to help them make some interpretations about the scale scores obtained.

Completing the Discharge Status Score Summary. This form (see Fig. 2) will allow you to see, at a glance, the number and percentage of clients discharged to each location and for each primary reason. Once the Quality Assurance Committee specifies the charts they want reviewed (e.g., 10 percent of all charts closed between specified dates), the records/clerical staff can pull the specified charts. If your professional staff have been completing a Discharge Status Scale on each client at the time they write their discharge summaries and have been including it in the client's chart, your records/clerical staff will only need to transcribe each client's chart number and discharge scores onto the Discharge Score Summary. If your professional staff have not been completing a Discharge Status Scale on each client at discharge, your records/clerical staff would need to review the chart and complete a Discharge Status Scale before transcribing the chart numbers and discharge status scores (discharge location and primary discharge reason) onto the Discharge Status Score Summary.

The records/clerical staff person would then count up the number of clients receiving each discharge location and primary reason for discharge score. They would also calculate the percentage of clients (of those charts reviewed) with each location and primary reason score.

Spaces have also been left for the dates of the review (i.e., the time frame during which the clients listed on the Score Summary were discharged) and the percentage of clients sampled. These data will facilitate your Quality Assurance Committee's record keeping of what charts were reviewed and when.

Using the Scale for Quality Assurance

The Number of Charts to Review. For quality assurance purposes, it is recommended the Quality Assurance Committee (or designates) within your agency randomly select 10-15 percent of your agency's closed charts for review.

When to Survey. As it is also being recommended that each agency review the discharge status of their clients at least twice a year but, preferably, once a quarter, your Quality Assurance Committee will need to explicitly state which charts are to be considered for selection. If you choose to review the discharge

FIGURE 2
Discharge Status Score Summary Form

DISCHARGE STATUS
SCORE SUMMARY

Date of Survey _____ _____
        (M/D/Y)   —   (M/D/Y)

% of Closed Charts Reviewed_____

	DISCHARGE LOCATION																	PRIMARY REASON FOR DISCHARGE												
CHART NUMBER	Client's Own Home - Lives Alone Without Referral	Client's Own Home - Lives Alone With Referral	Client's Own Home - Lives With Others Without Referral	Client's Own Home - Lives With Others With Referral	Family Member's Home - Without Referral	Family Member's Home - With Referral	Foster Care / Adult Family Home Without Referral	Foster Care / Adult Family Home With Referral	Congregate Care / Retirement Facility Without Referral	Congregate Care / Retirement Facility With Referral	Nursing Home	Acute Care Hospital	Psychiatric Hospital / Inpatient Substance Abuse / Certified Rehabilitation Unit	Expired at Home	Expired in Health Care Facility	Other		No Longer Homebound	No Longer Requires Skilled Care	Client / Family Can Manage Alone	Client / Family Refused Service	Admitted to Health Care Facility	Require: Type of Service Not Provided	Agency Has Insufficient Resources	Client / Family Has Insufficient Financial Resources	Continued Care Not Approved or Authorized by Physician	Continued / Prolonged Non-Compliance on Part of Client / Family	Moved	Expired	Other
	1	2	3	4	5	6	7	8	9	10	11	12	13	14	15	16		1	2	3	4	5	6	7	8	9	10	11	12	13
NUMBER																														
PERCENT																														

status of your clients twice a year, you would need to review the charts closed within the past six months.

How to Select Charts for Review. The easiest method of random chart review is to obtain a list of all chart numbers of clients discharged within the time frame you have selected and count the total number of chart numbers on your list. Determine the number of charts you will need to select to realize 10 percent (or 15 percent) of your sample. For example, if you want to review 15 percent of 200 clients discharged between December 1, 1985 and May 31, 1986, you will need to select 30 charts for review. Dividing 200 by 30, you will find you will need to select every sixth chart for review. Have your clerical staff person select a random starting point on his/her list of chart numbers, and go through the entire list pulling every sixth chart. Have them pull the charts and fill in a copy of the Discharge Status Score Summary. Once the Discharge Status Score Summary form is complete, the records/clerical staff person is to give the completed form to the Quality Assurance Committee for their review.

Interpreting the Data and Taking Action. By looking at the Discharge Status Score Summary, your Quality Assurance Committee will be able to see, at a glance, the percentage of surveyed clients discharged to each location and for each primary reason. An example Score Summary form—completed by one agency while pilot testing the scale—is included in this chapter (see Fig. 3).

Red flag areas of possible concern to your Quality Assurance Committee might be an excessive percentage of clients discharged to (1) the client's own home without referral, (2) nursing homes, (3) acute care hospitals and (4) expirations at home. At this moment in time, as no standards have been set, "excessive" discharges to each of the above locations can only be defined in terms of your Quality Assurance Committee's clinical judgement. After these data are collected for some period of time in your agency and you implement changes to positively impact your discharge location/primary reason scores, you will know what you are obtaining and what is feasible. At this time and based on these data, you can then set your own standards. For further information on standards, see the section entitled Setting Standards in the chapter on General Symptom Distress in the complete manual.

Looking at the sample of a completed Score Summary form (see Fig. 3), you will note that, of the charts reviewed, 40 percent of the clients were discharged to their own home without referral and 28 percent were discharged to an acute care hospital. This Association's State Quality Assurance Committee thought that both these figures would warrant further investigation to ensure the appropriateness of each discharge location. It is thought that each expiration at home should be investigated to ensure that the death was expected and planned. If unexpected, the chart should be reviewed to determine the circumstances of the death and to assure that the death was not related to what was done or not done in the process of care.

FIGURE 3
Sample Completed Discharge Status Score Summary Form

DISCHARGE STATUS
SCORE SUMMARY

Date of Survey 3/10/86 (M/D/Y) — 6/30/86 (M/D/Y)

% of Closed Charts Reviewed 24% OF ALL CLIENTS DISCHARGED DURING ABOVE DATES

DISCHARGE LOCATION

1. Client's Own Home - Lives Alone Without Referral
2. Client's Own Home - Lives Alone With Referral
3. Client's Own Home - Lives With Others Without Referral
4. Client's Own Home - Lives With Others With Referral
5. Family Member's Home - Without Referral
6. Family Member's Home - With Referral
7. Foster Care / Adult Family Home Without Referral
8. Foster Care / Adult Family Home With Referral
9. Congregate Care / Retirement Facility Without Referral
10. Congregate Care / Retirement Facility With Referral
11. Nursing Home
12. Acute Care Hospital
13. Psychiatric Hospital / Inpatient Substance Abuse / Certified Rehabilitation Unit
14. Expired at Home
15. Expired in Health Care Facility
16. Other

PRIMARY REASON FOR DISCHARGE

1. No Longer Homebound
2. No Longer Requires Skilled Care
3. Client / Family Can Manage Alone
4. Client / Family Refused Service
5. Admitted to Health Care Facility
6. Requires Type of Service Not Provided
7. Agency Has Insufficient Resources
8. Client / Family Has Insufficient Financial Resources
9. Continued Care Not Approved or Authorized by Physician
10. Continued / Prolonged Non-Compliance on Part of Client / Family
11. Moved
12. Expired
13. Other

CHART NUMBER	Discharge Location	Primary Reason for Discharge
3998	15	12
1164	2	13
1462	12	5
1500	1	3
1260	12	5
3230	2	4
0403	1	4
3277	11	5
3283	1	2
3973	1	3
1481	1	2
1527	12	5
1546	12	5
1556	2	2
1569	12	5
2610	1	4
3736	12	5
2624	1	2
4062	1	3
3892	12	5
1573	12	5
3149	2	2
1582	1	9
4036	1	2
1648	1	2

NUMBER — CONTINUED OVER

PERCENT — CONTINUED OVER

FIG. 3 (continued)

DISCHARGE STATUS
SCORE SUMMARY

Date of Survey 3/10/86 — 6/30/86
(M/D/Y)   (M/D/Y)

% of Closed Charts Reviewed 24%

DISCHARGE LOCATION (columns 1–16)

1. Client's Own Home - Lives Alone Without Referral
2. Client's Own Home - Lives Alone With Referral
3. Client's Own Home - Lives With Others Without Referral
4. Client's Own Home - Lives With Others With Referral
5. Family Member's Home - Without Referral
6. Family Member's Home - With Referral
7. Foster Care / Adult Family Home Without Referral
8. Foster Care / Adult Family Home With Referral
9. Congregate Care / Retirement Facility Without Referral
10. Congregate Care / Retirement Facility With Referral
11. Nursing Home
12. Acute Care Hospital
13. Psychiatric Hospital / Inpatient Substance Abuse / Certified Rehabilitation Unit
14. Expired at Home
15. Expired in Health Care Facility
16. Other

PRIMARY REASON FOR DISCHARGE (columns 1–13)

1. No Longer Homebound
2. No Longer Requires Skilled Care
3. Client / Family Can Manage Alone
4. Client / Family Refused Service
5. Admitted to Health Care Facility
6. Requires Type of Service Not Provided
7. Agency Has Insufficient Resources
8. Client / Family Has Insufficient Financial Resources
9. Continued Care Not Approved or Authorized by Physician
10. Continued / Prolonged Non-Compliance on Part of Client / Family
11. Moved
12. Expired
13. Other

CHART NUMBER	L1	L2	L3	L4	L5	L6	L7	L8	L9	L10	L11	L12	L13	L14	L15	L16	R1	R2	R3	R4	R5	R6	R7	R8	R9	R10	R11	R12	R13
1577	X																		X										
1592													X														X		
8109	X																										X		
8578				X																X									
8617	X																	X											
1563		X																X											
1501																X										X			
1505											X									X									
1086		X																											X
3006											X									X									
0323	X																		X										
9308		X																X											
4610																X											X		
1091	X																			X									
5285																X											X		
2350	X																	X											
6113												X									X								
2523												X									X								
NUMBER	17	7	0	0	1	0	0	0	0	0	1	2	0	0	1	3	0	1	7	3	3	0	0	0	1	0	3	3	2
PERCENT	40	16	0	0	2	0	0	0	0	0	2	28	0	2	2	7	0	26	16	7	30	0	0	0	2	0	7	7	5

If dissatisfied with a 40 percent discharge to own home without referral, the Quality Assurance Committee would need to determine what courses of action they could take to reduce this percentage (see section on Causes of Action in the General Symptom Distress Chapter in the complete manual), choose a course of action and implement it, and then retest several months later to see if the action reduced the percentage. If it has not been reduced, they would choose another course of action, implement it, and retest again.

Process-Outcome Studies. What is eventually required is some evidence of the link between what you do and don't do to/for/with your clients to realize the best discharge status possible. Once your review system is working smoothly, your Quality Assurance Committee can begin to investigate this link by examining the effects of various factors on discharge location. For example, perhaps more clients could be discharged to their own home or a family member's home if your agency improved their discharge planning—start it earlier, involve the family more, increase ties with other community resources. To check this out, the Quality Assurance Committee would need to hold an in-service on improving discharge planning—offering clear recommendations in terms of when it should be started, who is to be involved, etc. They could then check out the impact of this improved planning by using it with some current at-risk clients and not others, and then compare discharge locations.

Process-outcome studies are an important part of a quality assurance endeavor. Only by comparing clients with favorable and unfavorable outcomes and investigating for possible differences in the process of care will we begin to know what processes of care yield the best outcomes possible. Only by deliberately changing what we do for/to/with our at-risk clients and investigating the outcomes will we be able to establish the link between processes of care and client outcomes.

Reliability of the Scale

Interrater Reliability. Interrater reliability was established by having three staff (records/clerical and professional) independently complete a Discharge Status Scale on approximately 20 percent of the charts reviewed. The interrater reliability was found to be respectable: 83.3 percent for discharge location and 75.8 percent for discharge reason.

Based on feedback obtained by pilot site staff, the discharge locations, primary reasons, and accompanying instructions have been modified to clear up ambiguous areas. It is thought that the interrater reliability for this scale will now be higher.

Internal Consistency. Internal consistency is an inappropriate measure of reliability for this scale as discharge location and primary reason for discharge measure two distinct aspects of discharge status.

Test-Retest Reliability. As it is usually conceived—to test the stability of a scale over time—test-retest reliability is inappropriate for this scale. This test of reliability is usually used on constructs not expected to vary from time one to time two (e.g., intelligence). It is expected, however, that clients admitted and discharged from Home Care Service more than once will not always be discharged to the same location each time or for the same reason.

Validity of the Scale

Face Validity. Face validity was established by having the Home Care Association of Washington's Quality Assurance Committee rate the appropriateness of the scale for home care. The face validity of the scale was rated as being good (out of rating possibilities of poor, fair, good) by 100 percent of this State's Quality Assurance Committee. The face validity was also rated by the five home care sites who piloted this scale. It was judged to have good or excellent face validity by 78 percent of the pilot site staff who completed the evaluation forms.

Content Validity. Content validity involves the systematic examination of the scale's content to determine whether it includes a representative sample of the domains of discharge status, and whether the response categories represent the majority of possible home care discharge locations and primary reasons.

Content validity was assured by (1) examining the professional literature for discharge status scales and methodologies developed by other experts in home care and long term care; (2) having this Association's State Quality Assurance Committee and their agency staff help determine the discharge status possibilities for home care. The content validity of the scale was judged as good by 100 percent of this Association's State Quality Assurance Committee. Of the pilot site staff who completed the evaluation form on the scale, 77 percent thought the scale to be complete.

Construct Validity. Construct validity of the scale has been established. It was tested on 166 clients across five home care agencies within the state of Washington. The results of the analyses were compared against some preconceived hypotheses. For example, it was hypothesized that sex alone would not affect discharge location. This hypothesis was supported (F (1) = 3.55, p is greater than .05).

It was also hypothesized that age alone would not significantly affect discharge location, but the trend would be for older persons to be discharged to family home or nursing home. The data supported this hypothesis (see Table 1). The analysis did not show a significant effect (F (3) = 1.53, p is greater than .05) but the trend was in the correct direction.

TABLE 1
Clients' Discharge Location by Age

	Percentage of Clients Discharged		
Age	Own Home	Family Home	Nursing Home
20–64	60	7	0
65–74	72	12	2
75–84	62	10	7
85+	57	17	13

It was hypothesized that clients with multiple diagnoses (four or more) would be more likely to be discharged to places other than their own home than persons with 0 to 1 additional diagnoses. This hypothesis was also supported (F (1) = 4.66, p = .03).

It was hypothesized that client acuity would also affect discharge location scores: clients with low acuity (requiring only one visit every four or more days) would be more likely to be discharged home than clients with high acuity (one visit every day or more than once a day). This hypothesis was supported (F (1) = 4.19, p = .05).

It was hypothesized that clients with a primary diagnosis of mental disorder/confusion would be more likely to be discharged to places other than their own home than would clients with other primary diagnoses. This hypothesis could not be tested due to the small numbers of clients (N = 2) with this primary diagnosis.

ABOUT THE AUTHOR

Bernadette Lalonde, PhD, is Principal, Lalonde Research and Consultation, Seattle, Washington.

REFERENCES

1. The first edition of the manual is available for purchase from the Home Care Association of Washington, 406 Main Street, Suite 116, Edmonds, WA 98020 (tel. 206-775-8120) for $40 plus $5 shipping and handling. Two additional scales, Family Strain and Functional Status ($5 each) will be available in August 1987.